Hormonal Manipulation

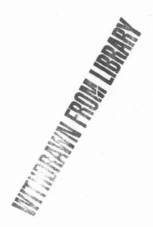

William N. Taylor, M.D.

Hormonal Manipulation

A New Era of Monstrous Athletes

McFarland & Company, Inc., Publishers
Jefferson, N.C., and London: 1985

Dedication

This book is dedicated to the children of my life: Nathan, Caroline and Ashley. In helping to guide them to happiness, I hope to discard the concept of the "American Dream" and instill in them the basis for happiness with whatever and whoever they wish to become. In this manner, I hope always to rate highly on their lists of best friends.

This book is equally dedicated to Susan P. Taylor, my wife, lover, and best friend. Together, we have shared so many ideas and events that it is difficult to determine where she ends and I begin; she has had more ideas "bounced off" her than a backboard. Therefore, this book contains many of our "rebounds."

Finally, this book is dedicated to my Mom and late Dad. Although my Dad was a professional baseball player in his youth and my Mom and Dad attended every sporting event I entered, they never pushed athletics on me to the point of overshadowing the other important facets of life. I will be forever indebted for their clairvoyance.

Front cover illustration by Thomas A. Elisii

Library of Congress Cataloging in Publication Data

Taylor, William N.
   Hormonal manipulation.

   Includes index.
   1. Doping in sports.   2. Hormones — Physiological effect.   I. Title.
   RC1230.T393   1985   615'.36   85-42523

ISBN 0-89950-166-4 (alk. paper)

Printed in the United States of America

McFarland   Box 611   Jefferson NC 28640

Table of Contents

Acknowledgments

I would like to specially thank the following people for their ideas, directive suggestions, and opportunities to meet most of the "players" involved with the anabolic hormone issue in sports:

Stan Heinricher, editor of *Nautilus* magazine;

John A. Lombardo, M.D., medical director of sports medicine, The Cleveland Clinic Foundation;

Ronald M. Lawrence, M.D., Ph.D., president and founder of the American Medical Joggers Association and finisher of 100+ marathons;

Richard T. Herrick, M.D., president of the United States Power-lifting Federation Sports Medicine Committee;

Jack H. Scaff, M.D., founder and annual finisher of the Honolulu Marathon;

John K. Robinson, M.D., associate dean of student affairs, University of Miami School of Medicine;

Arthur J. Pearl, M.D., orthopedic surgeon, Miami, Florida;

Kenneth Levy, M.D., orthopedic surgeon, Punta Gorda, Florida;

Terry Todd, Ph.D., world-class athlete and sports writer for *Sports Illustrated*;

Gary K. Buffington, M.D., chief of emergency medicine, West Florida Hospital, Pensacola, Florida;

Linda Schlumbrecht, M.D., president of Quik Care, Sarasota, Florida;

Robert Voy, M.D., chief medical officer, U.S. Olympic Committee;

Robert Goldman, D.O., sports medicine director, Chicago Osteopathic Hospital; vice president, AAU;

Richard Brown, head coach of Athletics West;

Richard Strauss, M.D., vice president of the American College of Sports Medicine;

James Wright, Ph.D., captain, U.S. Army.

Preface

This book is intended to provoke, to inform and to predict. It deals with the most controversial aspect of modern athletics: using extra doses of the body's own hormones to produce athletes with abilities far beyond those they would otherwise possess. Current estimates claim that more than a million fitness-oriented Americans are involved with the phenomenon of self-administering and self-experimenting with anabolic hormones to alter one or more facets of their athletic potential and physique. This phenomenon has expanded to become an international, interdisciplinary, and intergenerational dilemma with heavy financial and political overtones.

One of the major challenges of modern times is associated with culturing the inventions and technical advances created by human genius. Through recombinant-DNA genetic engineering techniques, the methods of modern genius have essentially taught bacterial cell cultures to synthesize many of the hormones which regulate the complex endocrine systems within the human body. The dilemma of how to use these fruits of genetic engineering has filtered its way into the athletic arena in a major fashion. It will also secure a major role in the practice of modern medicine, and may for many physicians represent the potential for extreme ethical backlash.

In the late 1700's, Alexander Hamilton said, "Men give me credit for genius; but all the genius I have lies in this: When I have a subject on hand, I study it profoundly." It is my intent that the pages which follow will contribute something of value toward a profound study of hormonal manipulation. Culturing human genius through profound study is what Alexander Hamilton (1757–1804) had in mind, and that concept was indoctrinated well over a century before man learned to culture bacteria!

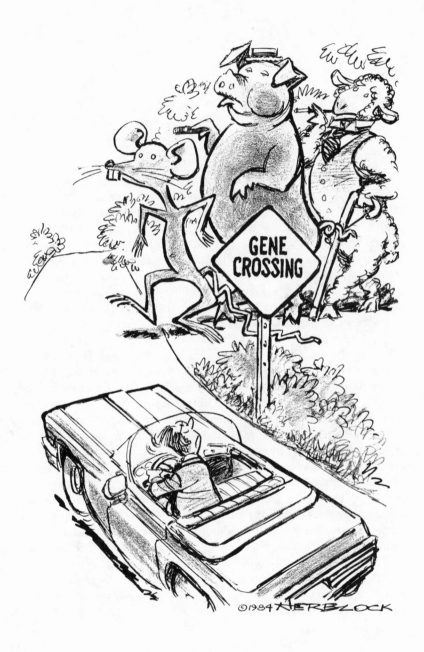

Introduction:
Culturing Human Genius

The hormonal manipulation of athletes essentially began well over a decade ago with anabolic steroids, which are powerful synthetic analogs of the male sex hormone, testosterone. The inventors of anabolic steroids had envisioned that these hormone analogs would be useful in treating many illnesses which afflict humans; but unfortunately, the initial clinical trials using anabolic steroids on a variety of poor health conditions were performed at a time when the investigational tools of medical science had not evolved far enough to accurately determine the full range of potential beneficial effects. In many cases, the effects of anabolic steroids on humans were so prominent that harnessing their potentials became a therapeutic problem. Subsequently, fewer medical studies using anabolic steroids were undertaken, and presently, only vague, ill-defined medical applications for using anabolic steroids exist for treating persons with diseased conditions.

Hormones such as anabolic steroids are powerful biological regulators of the intertwined bodily functions. In certain disease conditions, when a human lacks just a single hormone, the entire body declines, resulting in poor health, poor growth and development, and usually, early death. And, along these same lines, extreme excess of just a single hormone can cause devastating changes to the human body and mind.

During the past decade, five major concurrent events have taken place which will determine the ultimate fate of anabolic steroids and the effects which they have on humans. These events are:

(1) a decade-long drought for investigational research designed to study the effects which anabolic steroids have on humans, especially athletes;

(2) an exploding increase in the numbers of young fitness-oriented people who are self-experimenting with anabolic steroids without the proper medical knowledge or supervision;

(3) the advent of a variety of newly updated medical research tools which may be employed to ultimately determine the effects which anabolic steroids have on humans;

(4) the nearly exponential increases dealing with the financial gains awarded of late to athletes who excel in particular areas of sport;

(5) the progression of national and international political importance placed on athletic achievements.

Unfortunately, the constraints of time, and of the time lost by previous procrastination, will impede the scientific experiments which, if done properly, could have helped unravel some of the major aspects of the anabolic steroid dilemma. Historically, the consensus of the sports medicine platform on this issue rested firmly on the claim that anabolic steroids did not enhance athletic performance and to study them in athletes in the doses that the athletes were already taking would be dangerous. And, furthermore, any physician who wished to believe otherwise was confronted with the italicized statement in the *Physician's Desk Reference*:

> *WARNING: ANABOLIC STEROIDS DO NOT*
> *ENHANCE ATHLETIC ABILITIES*

For most physicians, tackling the issue through this meshwork of half-truths and outright untruths was not worth jeopardizing their entire medical careers, for which they had worked hard to achieve. But, many silent physicians truly believed that these drugs had some beneficial effects on some athletes. Some of these just simply resorted to prescribing anabolic steroids for their athletic patients without the proper supportive medical stands, dogmatic as they were.

The athletic arena, which was acutely aware that anabolic

steroids had powerful effects on athletic physique and performance, simply went underground for both the acqusition of the drugs and the hearsay knowledge which accompanied the purchase of the drugs. As the use of anabolic steroids became more prominent among athletes, so did the consequent measures for "cover up." These "cover ups" began to occur at all levels of athletic competition, and this phenomenon tended to give rise to a general consensus untruth from the athletic arena: "These reckless rumors of drug use among our athletes are overreacting to the degree of the problem."

For every athlete who is experimenting on himself/herself with anabolic steroids, and now with a variety of other anabolic hormones, there is a case-study. Even with the anecdotal nature of these thousands of case-studies, the sports medicine world had to begin to listen to the claims and observe the alterations in both the human physique and human performance aspects. Subsequently, because of the efforts of a few "reckless-abandon," open-minded sports medicine physicians, and because of the efforts of the numerous hormonally-manipulated athletes, a major trend has begun to form. Essentially, a trend towards accepting that anabolic steroids do enhance athletic abilities is occurring among some of the major sporting associations. However, this trend may be "too little, too late."

The ramifications of genetic engineering are thrusting with tremendous velocity into the athlete's world. Medical scientists have progressed to a point at which they can identify, isolate, and subsequently synthesize many of the major hormones of the body so quickly that even the scientists cannot begin to study the effects of these hormones on humans prior to their release on mankind. This is primarily due to the powers associated with private enterprise lobbying techniques. And, the sports medicine world is not even yet sure how to handle the anabolic steroid issue which is over a decade old! We simply do not have the luxury of a decade of time to determine which avenues mankind will take along the paths of the continuing saga of hormonal manipulation of humans.

So while the issues regarding the anabolic steroid situation as it deals with modern athletics continue to blossom and expand in magnitude, other anabolic hormones have been introduced onto the athletic scene. Furthermore, some of these other anabolic hormones have the potential, if used repetitively in physically immature humans, to alter significantly the complex factors which regulate human growth and development. These particular anabolic hormones have been identified, isolated, and synthesized in accordance with the principles of recombinant-DNA genetic engineering. The primary example of this is synthetic human growth hormone, but others, such as growth hormone releasing hormone and somatomedins which have recently been synthesized, are beginning to receive significant athletic attention.

As the ensuing parts of the book will indicate, the concept of hormonally manipulating athletes and children who will be the future athletes has evolved well beyond just that of the anabolic steroid controversy. This phenomenon is quickly becoming one of the first real, significant perils which has sprung from the scientific inertia fueled by genetic engineering. In effect, hormones, which have been intended for the betterment of unfortunate individuals afflicted with selected hormonal disorders, are finding their ways into the bodies of healthy athletes. And since the numerous self-experimenting athletes are accustomed to using powerful drugs, primarily anabolic steroids at this point, without the proper medical knowledge or supervision, then one may easily conclude that as other synthetic hormones are made available, legally or illegally, they will also traverse these, and future, athletic human bodies.

In the first parts of the book, the specific hormones and the pathways associated with these hormones will be presented from an athletic-interest point of view. In Part 6, several non-athletic, but similar, current methods of hormonal manipulation of humans will be covered. Hopefully, this will further place the hormonal manipulation of athletes into the proper perspective, for this is not the only area of human life where exogenous hormones are being used to alter human capacities.

Finally, in Part 7 the perspectives of all of the persons who are caught in this web of athletic-success-driven hormonal manipulation will be discussed. And, since the physician has traditionally been the responsible party for prescribing medications, a special section in this final part will address this ethical and moral bombshell which medical science under the auspices of somewhat blinded scientific inertia has dropped on the practicing physician with little prior warning.

Unfortunately, the "Golden Age" of medicine has given way to "modern medicine," and essentially two major things have happened to the practicing physician. First, with the ever-expanding responsibilities *and* liabilities placed on him, he has had a difficult time even "policing" his own area. Second, the general public has viewed the practicing physician with burgeoning disrespect of late due to the uncontrollable quest to legislate the limits of liability by the nation's lawmakers. Let this Introduction invite any who wish to legislate medical ethics and morals in this complex area of human endeavor, but only after reading the entire book. Then, if you have the appropriate answers, I am sure they must be heard, and soon!

> It would be naive to assume there are only benefits and no costs to the biological revolution.... We have to weigh the economic advantages of biotechnology against the possible adverse consequences for the future of civilization.... Genetic engineering opens up ominous new prospects. In nature, a sheep cannot mate with a goat. You cannot transfer genetic material from a human into the hereditary makeup of a mouse. If nature didn't provide these mating barriers, we'd have chaos. But, using the new techniques, genetic material from any species can be stitched together on a molecular level with another species. Science should not use these synthetic biological blueprints to create living novelties.... The biological revolution allows us to create forms of life that don't exist in nature. We'll increasingly be able to control living organisms by applying our own designing principles, and that raises fundamental social, environmental, ethical, and political questions unparalleled in history. Scientists should not be the only ones deciding issues that affect everyone on the planet. The courts can insure that the rest of us won't be left out of the debate.

> Jeremy Rifkin, President
> Foundation on Economic Trends
> October 1984

1

Anecdotal Anabolic American Athletics

Unheard-of strangeness in the quantitative proportions of bulk and substance is already apparent to modern philosophical scrutiny ... a loss of adaptability through the relative importance of bigness over variation.

H.G. Wells,
The Mind at the End of Its Tether (1946)

Introduction

Self-experimentation with anabolic steroids has become an insidious epidemic as the medical world takes steps to remove its head from the sand. This is the first in a series of parts on the concept of "selective gigantism."

Temptations today sometimes hide behind the auspices of seemingly good intentions, and for young fitness-oriented, athletically-inclined men or women, anabolic hormone use is this type of temptation. Therefore, the introduction of this part of the book will begin with a hypothetical situation which plagues thousands of moral American young men each and every year. For the sake of this hypothesis, the story will be entitled *It Happens Late Every Summer*.

Goldenboy was a proud member of the all-state high school football team his senior year of high school. And, shortly after the end of the football season, Goldenboy was approached by many college scouts who intended to sign him for a grant-in-aid for their college football program. He received several offers from major colleges to play, and since Goldenboy was close to his father and mother, he consulted them to help him make the selection of which college program to choose. After much deliberation, he finally made his decision, and he began to prepare for this outstanding opportunity. Throughout the remainder of the high school year, Goldenboy could not have been prouder, and neither could his father. His father was instrumental in starting Goldenboy in athletics with "pee wee" football, and his father never missed a game throughout Goldenboy's entire football career. He was there to talk to the physician when Goldenboy broke his clavicle and again when he broke his left arm during a game-saving tackle. Goldenboy felt obligated to excel in football to some extent, but he also had grown to love the game.

As the end of the summer approached, it was time to report to the college football program. Goldenboy had played both offense and defense in high school, but he was recruited to play defensive back by the college. As the early days of practice passed, the coaching staff began to realize that he was just a second too slow to play defensive back. However, Goldenboy was an excellent athlete, and the coaching staff began to feel that with a few "body dimension" changes, he would make an outstanding linebacker. However, he must add to his still-immature stature over 40 pounds of muscular bulk.

Quickly he became aware of the methods which the other players used to "bulk up." He didn't want to resort to using anabolic steroids, but considering all of the pressures he felt, taking the anabolics was the easy way out. Besides all the other players were on them, and he simply could not face his father if he failed to retain his scholarship.

So, in his first year away from home, Goldenboy had grown two inches and gained 40 pounds of muscular bulk. He also had grown somewhat distant from his parents, and he never told them about the anabolic steroids. Goldenboy was the product of hormonal manipulation, and he knew very little about the anabolic steroids except that they made him a better football player. He was stronger, bigger, tougher, more aggressive, less afraid, and healed from injury much quicker. What could be wrong with these drugs?

Anabolic Steroid Overview

In order to determine some of the effects of these drugs, it is necessary for the reader to understand this point: anabolic steroids do in fact enhance the performance and alter the appearance, size and psychological make-up of the athletes who use them. And the use of anabolic steroids by athletes may be serving as an impetus for the hormonal manipulation of future athletes in many ways.

Let's put this observation into a medical context. The growth and development of the human body is largely controlled by a complex network of molecules produced by some of the body's organs, and these molecules are known as hormones. Examples of hormones of this type are human growth hormone, testosterone and estrogen. Human growth hormone, produced by the pituitary gland, regulates many of the major metabolic pathways associated with human growth. The sex hormones, testosterone and estrogen, products of the testicles and ovaries respectively, determine the gender and sexual characteristics of humans. During the past three decades, medical scientists have discovered how many of these hormone molecules affect human growth and development — in both healthy humans and in people who are afflicted with certain diseases. One of the classes of molecules which have dramatic effects on the human body is that of steroid hormones.

The most common steroid hormones which are used in *healthy* people are the sex steroids, both of the female and male type. The female sex steroids, which are primarily estrogenic steroids, are used extensively in the birth control pill. The male sex steroids, which are the androgenic/anabolic steroids, are used extensively in modern athletics.

"Anabolic" means "to build" and anabolic steroids tend to increase constructive metabolic pathways within the body. Therefore, the anabolic steroids tend to make the body grow in certain ways. They are synthetic derivatives of the natural male sex hormone, testosterone. And, in effect, the anabolic steroids were made to mimic some of the bodily effects controlled by testosterone and to reduce some of the unwanted effects produced on the body by testosterone itself.

Since steroid hormones are such powerful molecules, once they are released from the organs into the bloodstream the body normally uses strict mechanisms to regulate their production and secretion. But when additional steroid hormones are introduced into the body by ingestion or injection, the normal balances and regulatory mechanisms may be altered temporarily or in some permanent but unpredictable fashion.

Several bodily functions are controlled directly or indirectly by testosterone. These functions are so varied that attempts have been made to classify them according to their androgenic and anabolic functions. This arbitrary classification scheme helps to define the theoretical differences between testosterone and its synthetic analog derivatives, the anabolic steroids. The anabolic derivatives tend to promote the anabolic functions listed below in Table 1 and to reduce the androgenic functions as well. However, the "perfect" anabolic (free of androgenic functions) steroid has never been discovered or synthesized.

Table 1: Comparisons of the Androgenic and Anabolic Functions of Testosterone in Men

Androgenic Functions

initial growth of the penis
growth and development of the seminal vesicles
growth and development of the prostate gland
increased density and pattern of body hair
development and pattern of pubic hair
increased density and distribution of facial hair
deepening tone of the voice
increased oil production of the sebaceous glands
increased sexual interest and desire
probable enhancement of the ability to think in abstract and
    spatial dimensions
various aspects of "male behavior" patterns

Anabolic Functions

increased skeletal muscle mass
increased organ mass
increased hemoglobin concentration
increased red blood cell mass
control of the distribution of body fat
increased calcium in the bones
increased total body nitrogen retention
increased retention of several electrolytes
increases in protein synthesis

Therefore, after scanning the variety of functions in which testosterone alters or controls, it is easily seen that this is a powerful hormone. However, the synthetic analogs of testosterone, the anabolic steroids, are similarly powerful, but they have been the least studied and least prescribed of the steroid hormones. Significantly more medical attention has been given to the study and use of the other steroid hormones — the corticogenics, estrogenics and progesterogenics. And, although at least a dozen supportive or secondary uses for anabolic steroids have been considered by academic and clinical physicians, *currently anabolic steroids have little primary purpose for the treatment of disease as defined by modern medicine.* Apparently, the overwhelming majority of anabolic steroid preparations go to athletes for the express purpose of enhancing athletic skills and parameters involved with their physiques.

Three major classes of anabolic steroids are currently available: (1) oral or sublingual tablets, (2) injectable oil-based liquids, and (3) injectable water-based preparations.

The oral anabolic steroid preparations continue to be the most popular with athletes today. These include Anavar®, Winstrol®, Dianabol®, Maxibolin®, Halotestin® and Adroyd®. The liquid forms, which are intended for intramuscular injection are DecaDurabolin®, Primobolin® and others.

Many serious athletes use two or more of the oral or the injectable preparations together, and in the athletic vernacular, this is known as "stacking." This use of several similar anabolic steroid preparations in moderate doses seems to further enhance some athletic skills and muscle growth, according to athletes.

Anabolic steroids are manufactured by over two dozen drug companies in the USA. Since the original patents for discovering many of these molecules have expired, generic copies of the drugs have become popular because they are much cheaper and highly available to the athlete. For instance, a small vial of the generic copy of Deca-Durabolin® may be purchased from a drug company for about $4, while the brand name product may cost nearly $20.

Federal law dictates that anabolic steroids in this country are available by prescription only, but several investigative surveys show that the majority of athletes obtain some or all of their anabolics *without* a legal prescription from a licensed physician. This non-physician source of anabolic steroids for athletic purposes has boomed in the past few years. A black market, in many areas it traffics in illegal "recreational" drugs such as cocaine and amphetamines. The number of athletes and "fitness buffs" who ingest unauthorized chemicals is impossible to determine, but there are probably over a million young people taking anabolic steroids self-experimentally. Flourishing alongside the black market supply of anabolic steroids is a selection of other prescription medications used by athletes to "treat" the so-called side effects that arise from taking moderate to high doses of the anabolic steroids.

The present predicament as to the ethical considerations of whether athletes should be permitted to use anabolic steroids didn't appear overnight. Several factors have contributed to the present complex problem. In the past decade, as information from properly and improperly designed studies indicated that anabolic steroids did indeed enhance some athletic skills even at relatively low doses, the major sporting associations discouraged further research. This occurred in the late 1970's and instead of funding going for athletic studies to determine the effects of the anabolic steroids, a major diversion in the monies went to support the elegant and expensive detecting equipment for discovering the anabolics in the body fluids of athletes. To date, the newer, sophisticated testing methods have not significantly halted the athletic use of anabolic steroids.

Furthermore, with little or no new reported medical literature on the athletic use of anabolic steroids to refer to, the clinical physician has only a shallow foundation from which to guide the young person embarking on an athletic career. So, in short, regarding this issue, modern medicine has been "caught with its pants down."

Recently, an isolated case of liver cancer and an isolated case of early heart attack in athletes who used large doses of anabolic steroids were reported in the medical literature. Did the anabolics cause this cancer and heart disease? No one can say for sure, but if there is indeed a cause-and-effect relationship, then it may be that we are entering the early stages of an epidemic. These isolated cases may just be the first of many cases, and since research on the effects of these anabolic steroids has been essentially halted, modern medicine is in a predicament regarding the prevention and treatment of these problems.

To conduct the proper research large sums of money must be available. But the lack of money has not been the only problem with this type of research on humans. The real problem is an ethical one: to document the long-term effects of anabolic steroids, human subjects must be used in properly designed studies for long periods of time. In earlier times, such research was performed on prison inmates, but this practice is no longer considered ethical. Therefore, it may be that when the arbitrators artificially halt needed research, this time can never be "made up." In other words, we need the results of the studies that should have been begun a decade ago, but were discouraged.

The mid-1970's also saw the appearance of some of the generic copies of the anabolic steroids. And, because of the proliferating black market distribution for these drugs, and at a reduced cost as well, a social trend arose: as athletes and other fitness-oriented persons who used anabolic steroids entered a cross section of the job market, they greatly influenced the image of fitness in this country.

Of great concern is the charisma of the recent wave of muscular people. Our children admire them, and most children would rather have a muscular body resembling those of a "He-Man" or other characters in "Masters of the Universe." In fact, in an informal poll of boys of ages three to five years conducted by me in my freestanding emergency center, over 50 percent of these young boys claimed to regard "Masters of the Universe" as their favorite television program! Adults, too, are becoming more accustomed to the appearance of highly developed human bodies. However, children, as well as most adults, are unaware that many of their heroes are addicted to anabolic steroids, and that without these drugs their imposingly muscular bodies would not exist.

In sports perhaps many outstanding performances would not also happen without chemical help from anabolic steroids. Often the difference between the mediocre and superior athlete may be attributed to the advantages afforded by the anabolics. These potential advantages include both mental and physical aspects. The potential physical advantages include increases in: muscular strength; muscle mass and size; storage of muscle glycogen; endurance capacity; blood volume; hemoglobin and hematocrit concentrations; healing rate of muscle, tendon and bony injuries; a general boosting of the immune system and reduction in body fat percentage and amount of sleep required. Potential mental advantages include increases in: desire to train and excel; tolerance to pain; energy level; aggressive behavior; mental intensity — all adding up to a significant "psychological high." With so many potential advantages to assist athletic performance, it is not difficult to understand why athletes use anabolic steroids.

Since prescribing of anabolic steroids to athletes remains legal, but ethically controversial, the majority of physicians avoid this practice. From this lack of practice, then, most physicians remain relatively ignorant in this area. Anabolic steroids are prescription drugs in the USA, and without a knowledgeable physician for the athlete to consult about the effects brought on by these drugs, the athlete generally gets misinformed.

This lack of accurate information has not halted the use of these drugs by athletes. An athlete typically observes a fellow athlete who has taken anabolic steroids and excels, so he probably considers them safe. Therefore, this situation is similar to the athletic version of "Three Blind Mice." In addition, the athlete usually believes that since he is taking the drugs, then it is his own personal business. So, he combines the lack of a legal, ethical avenue to obtain a prescription for anabolic steroids with their believed significant potential advantages, and naturally he obtains them on the black market.

This black market network poses some hazards to the health of the illicit drug user. Some athletes, who might use unsterile techniques in handling, relabel and repackage anabolic steroids and then sell them to friends. Add to this danger the habit of using concomitantly a dozen or more prescription medications to combat the side effects of "megadoses" anabolic steroids plus the risk that these drugs might cause some unforseen, long-term health damage, and the reader can see how competitive sports can produce the opposite of its well-being intentions. In many cases, parents introduce their children to athletics in hopes that this will dissuade the children from the peer pressures which tend to introduce their children to illicit drugs. Then, as it turns out, many of the better athletes use anabolic steroids and other drugs, which defeats the intended purposes for many parents. And, for the past few years, concerned people in high ranking positions are attempting to not only change the image of athletics, but to actually curb the drug use in sports. However, many of these initial attempts are failing, due primarily to the underestimation of the true problem.

Many people think that if all anabolic steroids were removed from the athletic world, athletes would have equal oportunities to excel and win. Certainly in nature this democratic sentiment is ignored. This is because every athlete has a unique response to the variety of training stimuli, and one of the more dominant factors in determining this response is the athlete's particular hormone balance. For instance, in men difference in the normal amount of testosterone in the blood can vary over threefold even among normal men. This considerable natural variance in male hormone levels predisposes men with high-normal levels to excel naturally in sports in which muscular strength and size are important. Also, thanks to the psychological effects of high levels of testosterone, and probably the synthetic analogs, these men may have advantages in areas of sports and other endeavors where mental intensity is important. Thus, in this way, Nature abhors "leveling." And, so does human nature, for the human desire to create new performance levels in all sports is paralleled by a much more pervasive undertaking—the science of biological genetic engineering. Researchers have learned to teach bacteria and some lower animals to produce human hormones within their non-human cells via recombinant-DNA genetic engineering techniques. Some of these anabolic hormones which are available now or that are on the forefront are synthetic human growth hormone, synthetic growth hormone releasing hormone, synthetic human somatomedin-C and others. These synthetic molecules are the major ones associated with the complex biological growth and development of humans, and as science marches ahead, the products of this type of human genius may predispose mankind and Nature, which both abhor "leveling," to make species of living animals, and perhaps some form of super-human, which would otherwise not exist. Therefore, the manipulative use of the body's hormones on itself, whether it be the decade-old anabolic steroids, or the forefront synthetic recombinant-DNA genetically-engineered hormones, is nothing short of the "Dr. Franken-stein" syndrome all over again.

Basically, there is nothing new in this type of impulse. For centuries animal breeders have competed to create the fastest thorough-bred, or the meanest pit bull dog by genetic lines, but now with hormonal tampering as well. Furthermore, this tendency in human behavior was noticed quite early in literature, and was symbolically depicted in the story of the Garden of Eden with its Tree of Life and humans who would be "gods" only if they would eat of certain "fruits."

Typically, it is assumed that athletes who excel do so by combining genetic potentials with personal desire, the ability to sacrifice and by following a finely-tuned training regimen. It is more difficult for people to accept that one athlete may excel thanks to the influence of selected drugs. But, as medical and scientific advancements continue, especially in the areas of anabolic hormones and their pathways in the body, athletic potential will not be determined by genetic factors alone. Depending on the state of medical ethics, soon the manipulation of athletes and future athletes by administering anabolic hormones may become the dominant factor in athletic excellence. What a pity!

No matter how much sand we have available for sticking our

heads in, the ethical and moral issues regarding anabolic steroid use in athletics must be addressed in a rational and factual manner. Determining the ethics and moral customs for our society is beyond the scope of the medical physician, especially when there is a relative lack of supportive, definitive medical knowledge on the subject. Ethical guidelines cannot be constructed in terms of society's best interests unless those who make the decisions are adequately informed.

Information should come from properly designed studies. But these may prove difficult to execute. For example, every best scientific experiment of this sort must have a control group—a number of subjects who would not be receiving the anabolic steroids. However, thanks to the marked physical and psychological effects of moderate to high doses of anabolic steroids, the group "on" the drugs would certainly become aware of their status rather quickly, and the control group, likewise, would realize that they were taking placebos. The athletic subject groups would have to be large enough to allow for statistically significant results, and careful selection of the subjects would have to be a primary feature of the design. However, even after all of the design problems are prospectively solved, long-term studies would almost require the selected athletes to give their bodies and lives to science. This is a difficult ethical dilemma.

Anecdotal Anabolic American Athletes

As previously mentioned, a conservative estimate as to the number of young Americans who are self-experimenting and self-administering anabolic steroids is at least one million. Athletes who self-experiment because of the various pressures and promised athletic rewards might be called "freaks" by some people. However, they are more accurately defined as normal products of hormonal manipulation, albeit self-induced. Could it be that over one million athletes are wrong about the beneficial effects on their bodies? Even if it means committing a crime to use them? To answer these questions, the believed beneficial effects and believed adverse effects must be examined.

Any drugs which are effective cause some adverse or unwanted conditions in some of the people who take them. With anabolic steroids, many of these adverse conditions seem to be dose-related; in general, the larger the dose, the greater the potential for the number and severity of these conditions to appear. For the discussion of the adverse potential conditions for anabolic steroid-using men athletes, it has been important to investigate both the psychological alterations and the physiological alterations separately.

Potential Psychological Alterations Induced in Men Using Anabolic Steroids

The understanding of the mechanisms in which hormonal imbalance induces or uncovers psychological conditions in humans is certainly in its infancy. However, in many cases, close longitudinal observations in men who cycle on and off anabolic steroids have provided information to fuel major concerns about behavioral changes.

There is no doubt that use of anabolic steroids, even in low doses, potentiates certain psychological behavior patterns in men. And, with men athletes who are using moderate and larger doses of anabolic steroids, total personality changes may take place, both while on the anabolics and after the anabolics are stopped. They definitely upset the man's mental network and psyche in a variety of sometimes unpredictable fashions. And, in many ways, the man athlete who cycles on and off of anabolic steroids may begin to possess two distinct personalities, both of which differ from the presteroid self.

Whether or not anabolic steroid use actually induces psychological changes in men athletes directly, or whether the anabolics just tend to uncover some of the underlying potential abnormalities is unknown at this time. In fact, both of these mechanisms could help account for the significant observed changes, especially in the heavier users. More likely, however, is that the anabolic steroids tend to cause a "shift" in the entire psychological balance within the man athlete. This "shift" tends to cause the normal mixture of psychological behavior to become polarized in a more hostile, aggressive, assertive nature so that ordinarily minor points of contention become intolerable situations which may ignite hostile and sometimes violent behavior. In this manner, seemingly moot points tend to become a nidus for inflammatory behavior. Therefore, this "shift" in psychological behavior induced by the anabolic steroids represents a major potential adverse condition which may result in devastating consequences for some athletes. Furthermore, in the perspective of a sports medicine physician who tends to have concerns regarding the "whole" athlete, it is important to evaluate whether or not this "shift" in behavior towards aggressiveness is not without drawbacks. In other words, many athletic events require "controlled aggressiveness" for success, and the man athlete will tend to deny that he has lost control of himself in non-athletic settings. So, for the concerned sports physician, it becomes a dilemma further complicated in that different men have differing capacities to "handle" the extra male hormones.

As previously stated, cycling on and off steroids, which may be a standard practice among athletes to circumvent some of the adverse physical effects, causes continual flux in the athlete's psychological balance. Some of the psychological changes commonly seen are contained in Tables 2 and 3 (see page 18), in regard to which it is important for the reader to realize the following concepts:

- that these psychological changes do not seem to occur in every man athlete equally;
- that in a given man athlete the observed changes seem to be dose-dependent to a significant degree;
- that these psychological changes represent a real threat to the interpersonal relationships of the athlete;
- that most men athletes will tend to deny or play down these psychological changes;
- that the positive effects which the moderate dose and greater doses of anabolic steroids may cause are not worth jeopardizing the athlete's psychological balance in most cases;
- that the athlete's body and mind must both be considered in the education processes for the potential risks and benefits;
- that the man athlete may tend to become addicted to the anabolic steroids because of the mental and physical changes he undergoes, and also never "come off" the anabolics to prevent these cyclic mental and physical changes the anabolics tend to cause.

The Steroid Spiral

There is likely to be a connection between the increased use of anabolic steroids in sports and the increasingly violent personalities of many athletes. Despite the reluctance generally associated with this topic, it behooves the young athlete to read of the psychological shortcomings of some of the sports heroes they are trying to emulate.

Hormones, such as anabolic steroids, are powerful regulators of complex bodily functions. In certain cases, when an otherwise

Table 2: Potential Psychological Alterations
Induced in Anabolic Steroid-Using Men

Alterations While on the Drugs

increased sex drive (libido)
increased appetite
increased aggressiveness
increased tendency for hostility
increased mental intensity
increased energy level
increased tolerance to pain
increased tendency towards "one-track-mindedness"
increased desire to train
increased tendency toward uncontrolled temperament leading to
    increased violence potential
increased tendency toward potentially violent sexual crime
increased self-esteem
increased ability to train with greater intensity
increased inability to accept failure or poor athletic performance
decreased tolerance level in general
increased tendency toward "explosive" aggressive behavior
decreased inhibitions for further drug use
psychological dependency for anabolic steroids
sleeping disturbances and nightmares

Table 3: Potential Psychological Alterations
Induced in Anabolic Steroid-Using Men

Alterations After Cessation of Drugs

decreased sex drive (libido)
decreased appetite
endogenous depression
decreased self-esteem
decreased desire to train
increased desire to again take the drugs
slowly improved ability to remain in control of behavior
decreased aggressive behavior
decreased tendency towards hostility and violence
slow return to usual sleeping patterns
decreased energy level slowly returning to a normal level
decreased mental intensity
increased tendency towards listlessness and apathy
decreased desire to train with intensity

normal human lacks just a single hormone, the entire body suffers disease; correspondingly, moderate excess of a single hormone can cause devastating changes to the human body and mind.

Anyone who reads sports news is aware of athletes' violent behavior both in and out of athletic settings. Often it seems inconceivable that the athletic "superstar" could be accused of such things as rape, spouse-beating, tavern fights, soliciting prostitution, armed robbery, illicit drug dealing and so on.

These largely denied and overlooked psychological alterations in the anabolic steroid–using athlete represent major sources for adverse conditions. The consequences of the more severe psychological alterations represent the worst "side effect" for many steroid–using men.

From the histories of steroid–using men, a definite pattern of behavior emerges: male athletes begin to take anabolic steroids in low amounts. They tend to cycle "on" and "off" the steroids over and over again. They tend to ingest and inject larger and larger doses on each cycle as they become more and more "masked" by these drugs. Their mood swings and subsequent behavior patterns widen until these personality changes violate others.

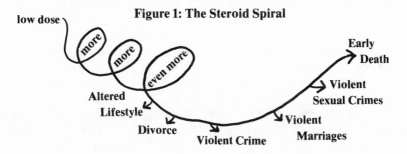

Figure 1: The Steroid Spiral

Potential Adverse Physical Conditions

Of all of the claimed physical disease conditions or abnormalities promoted to be caused by the prolonged use of anabolic steroids by athletes, liver tumors and cardiac disease seem to be the most severe. Many other less severe adverse physical conditions have been attributed to anabolic steroid use by both men and women athletes, and for the men, a lengthy listing of these less severe conditions will follow the presentation of the more severe ones. For the women, an entire part of this book is directed at this topic of concern.

Severe Liver Diseases
Associated with Anabolic Steroid Use

Apparently, two major forms of life-threatening diseases have been loosely attributed to the prolonged use of anabolic steroids: hepatocellular carcinoma (or liver cancer) and peliosis hepatis (or blood-filled sacs within the liver tissue).

The occurrence of liver cancer and other liver tumors in patients receiving anabolic steroid therapy has been the topic of several medical investigations. A summary from which this discussion is taken is contained in *Anabolic Steroids and the Athlete* (William N. Taylor; McFarland, 1982). As of 1978, 24 cases of tumors and tumor-like conditions of the liver have been reported in patients on prolonged therapy with anabolic steroids. Some of the interesting facts to be drawn from this summary of the literature are that:

- the dosages and length of therapy varied greatly; the average duration of the therapy prior to the discovery of the liver tumors was over 67 months of *continuous* anabolic steroid regimen therapy;
- over 75 percent of the cases were reported in patients with assorted anemias (or low red blood cell counts);
- over 50 percent of the cases were in patients who had received multiple blood transfusions;
- approximately 40 percent of the cases were reported in patients with Fanconi's anemia (which is a condition which has also been associated with many types of tumors including liver cancer even without anabolic steroid therapy) and;
- no cases were reported in otherwise healthy individuals, including athletes.

However, within the past year an isolated case of liver cancer was reported in the medical literature which was felt to be anabolic steroid induced in a relatively young athlete. This particular athlete claimed to have had heavy use of the oral anabolic steroids.

It is safe to say that moderate to heavy use of anabolic steroids in otherwise healthy athletes will cause liver cancer and early death in some of them. Which athletes will be ultimately afflicted with this dreaded disease is certainly unknown and unpredictable at this time. But, since the self-experimental use of these drugs has exploded in numbers and the amounts consumed and injected have skyrocketed within the past five years, it is to be expected that more athletes will indeed die from anabolic steroid induced liver cancer. Unfortunately, the time period from the initial stages of liver cancer on a malignant cellular level to the full-blown clinical expression of this killer may be more than five years. What this means is that there may be many athletes in this country right now with liver cancers growing in their livers, but the symptoms have yet to reveal themselves.

Certainly any athlete who has used enough anabolic steroids to be told that he/she is dying of liver cancer could address the issue of: ANABOLIC STEROIDS – WHY YOU DON'T NEED THEM! Especially, if this particular athlete never really made it big in athletics! As a warning then, do not assume that you will not be one of the athletes who is unfortunate enough to die a premature death owing to anabolic steroids obtained from a friend or black market distributor.

Peliosis hepatis is a rare condition consisting of blood-filled spaces in the liver tissue, and it is usually associated with tuberculosis or other wasting diseases. However, several reports have indicated that this condition may be seen in association with prolonged use of anabolic steroids. In the vast majority of the more than 20 cases reported, the patients had a severe hematological disorder or a malignancy (cancer) prior to the use of the anabolic steroids. The theoretical mechanism for this type of anabolic steroid related liver disease is essentially unknown, and no cases of anabolic steroid-using athletes have been reported with this disorder. Therefore, any assumption that anabolic steroid use induces peliosis hepatis in otherwise healthy athletes is essentially without basis at this time.

Severe Cardiac Disease
Associated with Anabolic Steroid Use

Heart attacks almost always result in the demise of young, muscular persons. Recently, Dr. O. Lynn Webb, a clinical physician in New Castle, Indiana, has shown that the athlete who uses moderate doses of anabolic steroids may be doing so at significant risk to his/her heart. Dr. Webb reported his findings at the 1984 annual meeting of the American College of Sports Medicine during a day-long meeting set aside to discuss drug use in sports. The measured blood lipid profiles which these athletes possessed have been equated with significant risk factors for early heart disease and heart attack. However, none of the athletes so far have proven to have clogged arteries shown by cardiac catheterization techniques. Even so, the high density lipoprotein cholesterol (HDL-C) levels, which are believed to be protective for the heart, were at least 50 percent lower when the athletes were "on" the anabolic steroids.

The apparently self-administered doses of anabolic steroids that the athletes were taking in this study were:

50–100 mg Dianabol® daily, plus
100–200mg testosterone cypionate by weekly injection, plus
100–200mg Deca-Durabolin® by weekly injections.

With the current knowledge regarding these changes in the lipid profiles, it has been estimated that this particular anabolic steroid regimen increases the risk of early heart disease and early heart attack by a fourfold factor. In some athletes, the residual effects of the anabolic steroid induced changes in the lipid profile persisted up to seven months after stopping the drugs.

It seems that there is strong evidence on the ability of moderate doses of anabolic steroids to potentially cause a heart attack in athletes by "sludging" the arteries which nourish the heart itself. This "sludging" is called atherogenesis.

If my theories, as well as others whom I have met with and trust their opinions and data, are correct, then the athlete who self-experiments with moderate to high doses of anabolic steroids along with the stresses associated with high intensity training, the stresses from peers, coaches and parents for athletic excellence, and who also use amphetamines and other stimulants along with extremes in dietary habits, may begin to fill our country's cardiac intensive care units. Therefore, it is my recommendation that all athletes take heed of this warning and reevaluate their anabolic steroid habit. Hopefully, if you are an anabolic steroid-using athlete, then you may live to thank me for this recommendation, for I believe that either you or some of your anabolic steroid-using athletic friends may die prematurely from cardiac disease which is anabolic steroid induced. In fact, I suspect that there have already been many cases of anabolic steroid induced heart attacks, but the persons afflicted with them either did not associate the possible connection between the anabolics and heart attacks, or they never lived to tell anyone about it.

Less Severe Physical Conditions
Associated with Anabolic Steroid Use in Men

Many of the common adverse conditions associated with the use of anabolic steroids in men, taken from *Anabolic Steroids and the Athlete* are listed below:

> hypertension or high blood pressure
> acne, both cystic and non-cystic
> fluid retention and edema
> mild abnormalities in liver function tests
> enlargement of the penis
> changes in libido (sex drive)
> nose bleeding
> viral illness after stopping the anabolics
> alopecia, or baldness of some type
> increased oil production in the sebaceous glands
> disturbances in sleeping patterns, nightmares
> increased appetite
> testicular atrophy
> decreased sperm count
> gynecomastia, or abnormal breast tissue
> deepening of the voice

Many of these adverse conditions are mild and reversible after cessation of the anabolic steroids, while others are irreversible. However, it is this list of pesky adverse conditions which may lead the anabolic steroid-using male athlete to polypharmacy, or using other drugs to combat these conditions. This topic will be discussed later in this part.

The Black Market Network for Anabolic Steroids

Obviously, anabolic steroids have to be manufactured and they must come from somewhere. Currently, they are manufactured by dozens of pharmaceutical companies in the U.S.A., some are manufactured and then subsequently smuggled in from other countries, and some are manufactured in "garage-labs" by ingenious individuals. Other primary sources for anabolic steroids used by athletes come from veterinary pharmaceutical companies, and the major anabolic steroids of this nature include Winstrol-V® and Equipois®.

After the drugs are manufactured, the major distribution network tends to exclude the legal avenue: the physician via a prescription subsequent to appropriate clinical procedures and examination of the athlete. However, a minor source of anabolic steroids used by athletes is indeed obtained in the legal manner above.

Many of the nation's health clubs and fitness centers are nothing short of drug stores for a wide variety of drugs, including anabolic steroids and other drugs used by athletes. Nearly every major health club or fitness center, even in some of the most remote cities, has someone actively selling and distributing anabolic steroids and other prescription drugs. And, since the health club and weight room techniques are encroaching on the training regimens of most sports, more and more athletes and fitness-oriented persons are coming in contact with this "drug store" phenomenon.

Other distribution sources of black market anabolic steroids include mail-order forms and promotional cards sent via the mail to a selected audience. Obviously, as the anabolic steroids and other medications change hands again and again, eventually they will end up in the hands of minors.

One of the major reasons that such an extensive black market exists for these drugs is that the penalties for doing so do not outweigh the financial gains, if indeed the illegal distributor is arrested and convicted. And, essentially, this area of illegal drug trafficking is no different than most of the illegal recreational drug trafficking, for not only are some of the "inspectors" involved with using the anabolic steroids themselves, but many of the "inspectors" may have financial rewards to "look the other way." After all, marijuana and cocaine are the major problems, aren't they?

A few of the major black market distributors who have confronted me over the past few years seem threatened by proposals to control anabolic steroid use. After all, this is how they make a living, by peddling drugs illegally. However, one suggestion, which I have made, that seems to cause some anxiety among these distributors is that of reclassifying anabolic steroids as scheduled drugs by the FDA. The major reason for this anxiety stems from the penalty for conviction which can be up to 20 years in prison.

Furthermore, since anabolic steroids are legal only via prescription means, the sports medicine physician's role in this matter is violated from the outset. In no other area of medicine is the physician confronted with healthy persons taking prescription medications without the consent of a physician. Furthermore, the athlete further violates the physician's role by asking him to "follow me, Doc, while I take the 'roids' and tell me that I am healthy."

Polypharmacy Associated with Anabolic Steroid Use by Athletes

Throughout the past decade of involving myself with athletes who use anabolic steroids as part of their training regimen, one of the more alarming, but consistent aspects associated with this use has been the use of other prescription medications. In many cases, the athlete who is taking high-dose anabolic steroids takes other medications, even more than most geriatric patients with total-body dwindling.

Before listing these drugs and classifying them further, it seems pertinent to present some concepts which surround this particular issue:

(1) As with the anabolic steroids themselves, most of these prescription drugs are obtained without a legal prescription from a licensed physician. In many cases, the local 'black market" distributors for the anabolic steroids also provide an access to the many other types of drugs frequently needed or used by the anabolic steroid-using athlete.

(2) Some of these medications have been used to "treat" some of the conditions which the use of anabolic steroids, especially in a dose-related fashion, seem to cause.

(3) Some of these medications have been used to augment even further the believed effects of the anabolic steroids.

(4) Some of these medications have been used to "treat" some of the minor injuries usually associated with strenuous athletic training.

(5) Some of these medications, especially amphetamines and diuretics have been used to reduce body weight prior to "weigh-in" periods for a particular event.

A complete listing of all of the drugs which have been used by anabolic steroid-using athletes is impossible to compile; however, an extensive listing will be included in the following table.

Table 4: Polypharmaceutical Drugs Usually Combined with Anabolic Steroids

Drug	Type of Drug	FDA Schedule
Nolvadex®	anti-estrogen	uncontrolled prescription
Clomid®	fertility drug	uncontrolled prescription
Fastin®	amphetamine	Schedule 4
Preludin®	amphetamine	Schedule 3
Didrex®	amphetamine	Schedule 3
Eskatrol®	amphetamine	Schedule 2
Trisoralen®	tanning pill	uncontrolled prescription
Oxysoralen®	tanning pill	uncontrolled prescription
thyroid hormone	hormone	uncontrolled prescription
amino acids	growth hormone releasers	non-prescription
caffeine	stimulant	non-prescription
diet pills	stimulant	non-prescription
codeine	pain reliever	Schedule 3
marijuana	recreational	Schedule I
cocaine	recreational	Schedule I
Indocin®	anti-inflammatory	uncontrolled prescription
Minocin®	antibiotic	uncontrolled prescription
Accutane®	anti-acne	uncontrolled prescription
Lasix®	diuretic	uncontrolled prescription
Aldactazide®	diuretic	uncontrolled prescription
Bumex®	diuretic	uncontrolled prescription
Halcion®	hypnotic	Schedule 4
Valium®	anti-anxiety	Schedule 4
Restoril®	hypnotic	Schedule 4
Xanax®	anti-anxiety	Schedule 4
Flexeril®	muscle relaxer	uncontrolled prescription
human growth hormone	hormone	uncontrolled prescription
glucagon	hormone	uncontrolled prescription
L-dopa	neurotransmitter	uncontrolled prescription
Catapres®	anti-hypertensive	uncontrolled prescription

It would be ludicrous to claim that *all* athletes who use anabolic steroids for their performance-enhancing potentials also used
numerous other prescription drugs. Obviously, many athletes may
probably use some low-dose anabolic steroid regimens without significantly adverse effects enough to resort to using other medications
to alleviate these adverse conditions. In other words, there probably
exists a regimen consisting of low-dose anabolic steroids which would
allow the athlete to avoid many of the more pesky adverse conditions,
but for several reasons, these low-dose regimens seem to now be far
removed from the moderate-dose and high-dose regimens currently
used by the majority of athletes today.

One of the primary factors which is reviewed when the FDA
classifies or reclassifies a particular class of medication is the potential for the class of drugs in question to potentiate further drug use.
Polypharmacy simply refers to the use of many drugs, and indeed, this
polypharmaceutical aspect of anabolic steroids is of major concern at
this time. And, after reviewing the diary material and personal habits
of hundreds of anabolic steroid-using athletes, I feel that the concerns about the use and misuse of other drugs along with the anabolic steroids makes for a very difficult situation, especially when an
athlete approaches me in my office, by letter, or by phone to discuss
his health care and health problems. And, I am not sure that this practice of using medications to combat the adverse effects of the initially
used medication is beneficial to anyone. It sure seems a long way from
the concepts of life-fitness and health with strength!

Anabolic Steroids Can Enhance
Athletic Skills and Performance

Recently, the American College of Sports Medicine altered its
position regarding the efficacy of anabolic steroid use in athletes by
now claiming that the use of anabolic steroids seems to enhance performance by influencing parameters in some athletes who are under-
going concomitant resistance training. This represents a *major*
change in the College's position, and it evolved essentially without any
significant changes in the reported scientific literature on trained
athletes. Therefore, to present the reported studies with trained athletes in regard to strength and muscular size, the following Table 5 (see
page 28) is included. This table represents a "rehash" of the available

Table 5: Summary of Anabolic Steroids Studies with Trained Male Subjects

Reference	Year	Drug and Dosage	Double-Blind Study	Cross-Over Study	Placebo Control	Protein Suppl.	Significant Increase in Mass/Strength	Statistically Significant Results
O'Shea & Winkler	1970	Anavar 10mg/day for 6 weeks	no	no	no	yes	yes	yes
O'Shea	1971	Dianabol 10mg/day for 4 weeks	no	no	yes	yes	yes	yes
Bowers & Reardon	1971	Dianabol 10mg/day for 5 weeks	yes	no	yes	yes	yes	yes
Ariel	1972	Dianabol 10mg/day for 8 weeks	yes	no	yes	no	no	no
Ward	1973	Dianabol 10mg/day for 4 weeks	yes	no	yes	no	yes	yes
Golding	1974	Dianabol 10mg/day for 12 weeks	yes	no	yes	yes	no	no
Stanford & Moffat	1974	Dianabol 20mg/day for 4 weeks	yes	no	yes	yes	yes	yes
O'Shea	1974	Winstrol 8mg/day for 4 weeks	yes	no	yes	yes	yes	yes
Berg & Keul	1974	Deca-Durabolin 50mg every 12 days for 8 weeks	yes	yes	yes	yes	yes	yes
Freed et al.	1975	Dianabol 10mg/day or 25mg/day for 6 wks.	yes	no	yes	no	yes	yes

(From William N. Taylor, M.D., *Anabolic Steroids and the Athlete*, McFarland, 1982) literature on trained athletes prior to 1982, and when the conclusions are placed in a table such as Table 5, it becomes evident that anabolic steroids taken in relatively low doses for short periods of time by men who are actively training have positive effects on muscular strength. However, a more careful examination of this table will reveal that the doses used by the athletes in these studies tend to be well below the actual doses consumed and injected by athletes today. And, the medical and scientific literature lacks the information that has probably the most practical value—how do the higher doses of anabolic steroids affect athletes? To search for the answers to this inquiry, it is necessary to observe and study athletes who have taken or are taking large doses, which can easily reach ten to fifty times the amounts used in the published literature.

Essentially, the effects of large doses of anabolic steroids on muscle mass and muscular strength are easily detected by the human eye, especially if these large doses are used by the athlete for three consecutive months or more. The muscular size increases of athletes using anabolic steroids in large amounts along with strength training regimens can be enormous when compared with the gains of athletes who train in a similar manner but without chemical help. In other words, these changes do not require the aid of a microscope, elaborate blood-testing or precisely calibrated strength-testing equipment for detection. In most cases, if valid information about the actual quantities of anabolic steroids taken by athletes is obtained, then observing the changes in muscular size and strength is no chore.

Bodybuilder's Syndrome

Most serious bodybuilders use anabolic steroids as a major part of their training, especially if they are competitive bodybuilders. The majority of them will "talk" anabolic steroids to a knowledgeable person, but usually only after they repeatedly deny the inquiry. Therefore, a superficial glance to determine the problem faced by many serious bodybuilders reveals very little information. But to those persons with an "in," a deeper look into the lifestyle of competitive bodybuilders reveals common patterns of significant physical, psychological and social problems, if indeed they are "chemical" bodybuilders.

When today's top bodybuilders began strength-training years ago, there were few highly developed models to emulate. In the mid-1970's, however, increasing numbers of bodybuilders began self-experimenting with anabolic steroids. Their dosages soon sky-rocketed, and up to a point, the more anabolic steroids they took, the greater the changes they noticed in their appearances and body sizes.

In general, most men who are now competitive bodybuilders have changed physically and mentally since their initial days of strength training. No bodybuilder will deny the physical changes, but the drug-induced psychological alterations are difficult for them to admit. Many of them have gone through a complete lifestyle meta-morphosis.

As many of these men began to reflect on their experiences and to share these experiences with others, they realized that they were actually "hooked" on anabolic steroids and the other drugs they had used along the way. The majority of these competitive bodybuilders had become chemical "junkies," and their hunger to discover and consume newer and better anabolic agents became insatiable.

Psychological addiction wasn't the only ground for further self-experimentation, for growing more muscular; they began to be selected by wealthy sponsors for posing and for advertising an assort-ment of products. Some of the "chemical" bodybuilders soon became wealthy themselves. However, many of them ignored and denied the psychological and social deterioration in their lives. They ignored, but usually paid the consequences for, the aggression and violent tempers which seemed to ignite everyone around them. They laughed at the 3:00 a.m. trips to the refrigerator for a large snack, and this soon became habitual.

Bodybuilders have tended to de-emphasize the sometimes insat-iable sexual drive, the extreme fluctuations in mood, the continuous bouts of acne, the marital problems and almost every other change they experienced. For many "chemical" bodybuilders, bodybuilding became a lifestyle obsessing them into "one-track-mindedness."

Mirrors began to plague them, for hours of posing in front of them is a critical aspect necessary for competitive bodybuilding. Eventually, the forerunner bodybuilders who began experimenting on low-dose anabolic steroids found themselves psychologically and physiologically dependent on large doses of these drugs. Without them, they could not maintain the physique which meant so much to them. And, instead of cycling on and off the anabolic steroids, the competitive bodybuilders began to stay on them longer and longer to the point of never stopping.

There were other compelling reasons for this phenomenon. The psychological "high" which the anabolic steroids afforded gave way to a sometimes severe depression when the drugs were discontinued. The insatiable sexual desire turned into its opposite. Instead of the large gains in muscle mass and strength, there were losses in mass and strength and the "plateau-ing" effect which seemed eternal. Invariably, "chemical" bodybuilders would experience significant signs and symptoms of immunological depression upon cessation of the anabolic steroids, and sometimes severe viral infections, or recalcitrant fungal infections would result. Also, the desire to train as they had while they were on the drugs seemed to evaporate. Many of the "chemical" bodybuilders who attempted to train strenuously while "off" of the anabolic steroids had persistant tendinitis and an occasional complete tendon rupture.

Many men who had extremely strict workout regimens while on the anabolic steroids would find themselves aimlessly walking about the gym floor, picking up a weight or two. Instead of nearly fighting with another bodybuilder who interrupted his workout program by using the same equipment, the bodybuilder "off" the anabolic steroids tolerated the perceived intrusion. The gym turf that once was worth fighting for, no longer seemed to be important. Stopping the drugs makes all the difference, but as many "chemical" strength athletes will relate, they have a difficult time staying off the anabolic steroids without a significant change in lifestyle or without resurrecting some old parts of themselves.

Everything in the world of bodybuilding reinforces pill-popping and intramuscular injections. The sponsorship money paid to the elite for posing and advertising has attracted increasing numbers of young people into the fitness arena. Many top bodybuilders, who know that their physiques are *impossible* to attain without the powerful effects of the anabolic steroids, mislead young people by attributing their success to other factors, which they know have little or no effect. Thereby, the former "gym rat" can become a successful businessman. This phenomenon now forms the basis for the lucrative bodybuilding industry. And, an ever-growing percentage of young athletes of all kinds are entering into the world of self-experimentation with anabolic steroids, and perhaps other newly synthesized anabolic hormones.

Summary: Anabolic Steroids Should Be Controlled Substances

In this part of the book, the material has been presented for the express purpose to indicate to the reader that anabolic steroids meet many, if not all, of the usual considerations that many other controlled substances have. By controlled substance, I mean that the U.S. Food and Drug Administration (FDA) has placed the class of drug in a category which allows for more specific control of the medication. With any controlled substance, such as narcotics, amphetamines, and various illicit drugs, the control of the medication is maintained by a variety of mechanisms. The degree of control usually depends on the summation of several parameters, and essentially, the control of the medication takes place every time the drug is dispensed from one location to another. Records which account for the dispensing information of every vial and pill of a controlled substance, must be kept. Drug Enforcement Agency (DEA) numbers must accompany orders from pharmaceutical companies or licensed physicians and research scientists. Also, knowing that these records are indeed kept, the people involved with the dispensing generally use more discretion with dispensing and prescription writing of the controlled substance. Therefore pharmaceutical companies and their representatives, pharmacists and physicians, are under greater obligation when controlled substances are employed. Also, the penalties for violating the laws and ethics which involve controlled substances are usually much stiffer for the convicted person compared to the penalties for uncontrolled substances. This deterrent effect can sometimes be instrumental in dismantling a well-developed "black market" network for illegal drug distribution.

General guidelines usually followed for placing a class of drugs into a controlled category include some of the following parameters:

(1) psychological dependency
(2) physical dependency
(3) abuse potential
(4) potential for leading to polypharmacy
(5) potential to reduce inhibitions for further drug use
(6) potential to potentiate use of controlled substances
(7) potential "black market" distribution patterns

(8) potential to potentiate underlying psychological tendencies and violence
(9) potential for "filtering" down of the drugs to children
(10) ability to cause potentially dangerous health risks.

In the preceding sections, a significant presentation of material on the points delineated above regarding anabolic steroids has been included. Anabolic steroid use by athletes without the proper medical supervision has the potential to result in all of these very serious situations. And, in my opinion, *anabolic steroids should be reclassified as controlled substances by the FDA.* Otherwise, the drugs just as well be non-prescription drugs so that anyone can have access to them.

The year 1985 may well bring one of the most staggering chapters in organized athletics: *the exposure of the anabolic steroid epidemic.* No sporting fan will be untouched. The irony is that it comes hard after the greatest triumph (in 1984) Americans participating in the Olympic Games have ever had.

Anabolic steroids were apparently first used in World War II; steroids were said to have been administered to Nazi SS troups in order to make them more aggressive and less fearful of violence. It has been speculated that these early anabolic steroids were used by Hitler and his entire military staff, which may have accounted for, in part, the "driven," aggressive and violent acts committed by the German military.

Shortly after World War II, anabolic steroids were administered to survivors of concentration camps for their potential protein and muscle-building properties. Today, the use of anabolic steroids is widespread in some Third World countries as "appetite stimulators"; however, it could be that these drugs are "feeding" the continued violence in these countries.

So, from my expertise, it seems that anabolic steroids, which seem to have a major *constructive* influence on the human *body*, have overwhelmingly *destructive* influences on the human *mind*, which may lead young, muscular, athletic men to have violent and irrational behavior. In this manner, then, "anabolic," which means "to build," is a misnomer.

2

Athletic Women and Anabolic Steroids — Androgynous Antipathy?

(Written with Susan P. Taylor, RN, BSN)

> As our minds have probed more and more curiously into the space-time continuum in which the drama of evolution has been framed, they have discovered one paradoxical aspect after another behind the plausible face of normal being.

> H.G. Wells,
> *The Mind at the End of Its Tether* (1946)

Introduction

The syndrome of "androgynous antipathy" has jolted nearly every modern sports enthusiast, especially of late. Essentially, the "androgynous antipathy" syndrome is defined as an inherent aversion or repugnance to the "hermaphroditic" athlete who has obvious characteristics of both sexes. However, to much dismay, the Barr body chromosomal tests performed on the buccal mucosa of these athletes reveals that they are of the female gender!

Concurrent with the above writings of H.G. Wells, Aldous Huxley wrote in the foreword to *Brave New World*: "The Brave New

World is not the advancement of science as such; it is the advancement of science as it affects human individuals. The triumphs of physics, chemistry and engineering are tacitly taken for granted.... It is only by means of the sciences of life that the quality of life can be radically changed. The sciences of matter can be applied in such a way that they will destroy life or make the living of it impossibly complex and uncomfortable; but, unless used as instruments by the biologists and psychologists, they can do nothing to modify the natural forms and expressions of life itself."

Today, many women athletes are "used as instruments" by the biologists and psychologists under the auspices of sports medicine physicians, sports psychologists, sports physiologists, athletic trainers, athletic coaches, overzealous fathers, boyfriends or husbands, as well as the wide variety of financial sports marketeers. One of the methods to "calibrate" the athletic women as "instruments" is via the use of anabolic steroids and other anabolic hormones, again under the auspices of winning at all costs. And, as the contents of this part will discuss, these women athletes who are indeed "instruments" have had and will continue to have their "natural forms and expressions of life" modified. In many ways, this modification of the natural form is permanent to both the body and mind, and perhaps the soul as well. This modification of the natural form may "destroy life or make the living of it impossibly difficult and uncomfortable."

Even in this era of women's rights and thrusts for equality, the woman and man who work side by side with the same job and job title have a relatively large differential in pay scales. Whether she is a physician, lawyer or common laborer, the woman makes only three-fifths what her male counterpart does. And, it has been projected that this differential in pay will persist into the 21st century.

Athletic achievement has traditionally offered some people an avenue away from the majority of oppressive factors. Athletic achievement also offers this relief from oppression rather quickly, unlike many of the more structured educational and business opportunities. Therefore, many women athletes are very vulnerable to any persuasion which offers a promise of subsequent athletic success. But in my opinion, most of the women athletes who use anabolic steroids to obtain their athletic success are just trading one form of oppression for another. And the woman athlete who reaches athletic success with the aid of anabolic hormones is promoting drug use to fellow competitors and future athletic women in the worst way.

The widespread use of anabolic hormones in women athletes

will ultimately jeopardize the success of women's athletics. In this way, "the sciences of matter can be applied in such a way that they will destroy life," particularly the life of athletics. For many men and women sports followers, the anabolic steroid induced "androgynous antipathy" is difficult to overcome. There is just no doubt that the women athletes who look like and act like their male counterparts are changing and jeopardizing the future of women's athletics. And this is just at a time when women's athletics is gaining some of the respect which it deserves.

For the future Olympic Games, the widespread use of anabolic steroids and other synthetic anabolic hormones, especially in women athletes, will tend to alter these games into a circus, with the spectators scurrying around to get a peek at the freaks. It may follow then that the majority of even the strongest and wealthiest sports enthusiasts will begin to see that there is more to life than athletics. Finally, if the pendulum indeed does swing back away from drug-induced athletic champions, then humanity will have surely made a monumental stride ahead.

Understandably, the quotes from the most famous science fiction authors are not true science. However, in many cases, the fictional aspect of science fiction is derived from within a framework of educated speculation coupled with an innate ability to understand human nature. So it is my intent that the reader keep the major emphasis of this introduction in mind as some of the current science regarding the athletic use of anabolic steroids by women athletes is presented. And, then, in the summary of this part, some additional philosophical points will be addressed concerning this topic of pervasive importance.

Medical Indications for Anabolic Steroid Use in Women

To date, the use of anabolic steroids in women athletes has never been studied by any formal investigational research group. However, there are some current medical indications for the use of these male hormone derivatives in women with selected health disorders. Most of these medical conditions will be listed in the following paragraphs of this text, along with a brief explanation describing some of the reasons for this type of therapeutic modality.

• *women with post-menopausal osteoporosis.* Post-menopausal osteoporosis is a degenerative condition in which a slow, steady amount of calcium is lost from the bones of the body and is greatly accelerated by the onset of menopause in women. This calcium loss, which may exceed 5 percent per year in some women, weakens the strength integrity of the skeleton and sets the post-menopausal women up for serious, sometimes crippling, fractures subsequent to the insult of even minor traumatic conditions. In many cases, in elderly women who have not had some type of hormonal replacement for several years, a hip fracture may usher in a sequence of events that end in a lengthy, devastating nursing home existence culminating in death due to the inability to ever ambulate efficiently again. Recent national estimates for the annual treatment of the conditions resulting from post-menopausal osteoporosis have ranged as high as four billion dollars.

When a woman reaches the menopause, her female hormone levels, especially the serum estrogen levels, reduce dramatically. And, in one sense, the post-menopausal woman becomes a hormonal neuter. This becomes an important factor in the pathogenesis of post-menopausal osteoporosis, for it is imperative, for reasons which are not fully understood, that the body's calcium balance is significantly intertwined with the existing hormonal balance. So, in effect, when a woman reaches the menopause her serum estrogen levels generally remain markedly reduced throughout the remainder of her life, and she is destined to lose skeletal calcium on a steady basis year after year until the bones are so brittle that they fracture due to minor trauma and have very little subsequent capacity to heal. And with the continual shift in most modern countries toward an aged population explosion, this condition is of paramount importance.

The majority of treatment modalities for post-menopausal osteoporosis have centered around estrogen replacement and calcium supplementation to the diet. This type of replacement therapy seems to slow, but not halt, the progressive loss of skeletal calcium, and there are major risks to the woman who selects estrogen replacement as her course of action. Some of these risks involve increased chance for cancer in the female organs, hypertension, strokes, liver disorders, mental instability, weight gain, fluid retention and thrombophlebitis. However, at this time, estrogen replacement, coupled with supplemental dietary calcium and exercise is the most generally accepted form of treatment.

At this time, the only form of therapy which actually *reverses* the calcium loss in the post-menopausal woman is cyclical treatments with low-dose anabolic steroids. Several scientific studies have pointed to the effectiveness of using low-dose oral anabolic steroids in the preventative and curative treatment of post-menopausal osteoporosis. And from these few reported scientific studies, it may be concluded that the benefits of low-dose anabolic steroids in some women with post-menopausal osteoporosis greatly outweigh the risks.

• *athletic women with amenorrhea.* As the competitive intensity levels continue to rise in women's athletics, so does the incidence of athletic amenorrhea, which is essentially the cessation of menstrual cycles in fit women athletes. This condition has been the topic of many investigational studies, but the exact causative set of circumstances which results in amenorrhea in a given woman athlete is unknown at this time. Several theories coupled with substantial supportive evidence suggest that there is a critical amount of body fat necessary for the woman to sustain normal regular menstrual cycles.

Recently, it has been reported that the woman athlete who has athletic amenorrhea tends to lose skeletal calcium at rates which approximate that seen in women with post-menopausal osteoporosis. In fact, the rate of skeletal calcium loss is as great as the most degenerative phases of post-menopausal osteoporosis. To date, this has been the most significant finding which suggests that athletic amenorrhea is indeed a potentially serious hormonal imbalance condition. And, as with the treatment of post-menopausal osteoporsis, low-dose anabolic steroid therapy in women afflicted with athletic amenorrhea could prevent some serious subsequent pathological fractures and "over-use" stress fractures which intense athletic training may produce. However, absolutely no scientific studies have been undertaken to study this potential use of anabolic steroids for women athletes.

• *women with endometriosis.* Endometriosis is a condition in which a speculative hormonal imbalance causes a chronic infectious process in the inner lining of the woman's uterus. The circumstances which cause this condition in any given woman are not fully known. It is usually considered that the basis for this condition usually has an underlying endocrine factor. For women in the childbearing years, endometriosis is a condition which can result in the inability to procreate.

The most successful treatment of endometriosis has come from the use of Danocrine®, which is a steroid molecule which has a mixture of endocrinological effects on the woman's body. It has a molecular structure most similar to Winstrol® which is an anabolic steroid in popular use by athletes. However, Danocrine® has been promoted as having a highly selective degree of anti-gonadotropin activity and its potential to cause anabolic and androgenic changes in women has been overlooked to a great extent.

Women afflicted with endometriosis should be educated to the potential adverse effects of Danocrine® therapy, including:

mental instability and changes in their psychological profiles,
virilizing changes in their faces, abnormal facial hair, and acne,
irreversible deepening of the voice,
irreversible enlargement of the clitoris, and
the potential to procreate a child with ambiguous genitalia.

Therefore, it is safe to say that in many ways, Danocrine® is an anabolic/androgenic steroid in women.

• *women with various anemias.* Anemic conditions in women can occur from a wide variety of circumstances, some of which may be ultimately diagnosed or remain idiopathic without detectable cause. Since anabolic steroids have been repeatedly shown to boost the immune system in general and stimulate the bone marrow to produce more red blood cells, they have remained part of the medical armamentarium for the treatment of various anemic conditions, especially when the anemic condition fails to respond to other therapeutic recourses.

• *women with various cancers.* Some of the major consequences and complicating factors seen with persons with malignancies are the dramatic catabolic responses, muscle wasting and prolonged anorexia. Furthermore, these poor health conditions are generally augmented by the treatment modalities such as chemotherapy, surgery, and radiation therapy.

Anabolic steroid treatment in conjunction with the other oncological therapeutic options has been used for years by some medical oncologists with some success. However, partially due to the prevailing medical antipathy of using male hormones in women for any reason, this use of anabolic steroids in women has been limited. However, if a certain drug has another major function in the body besides its anabolic potentials, it generally has avoided the repugnancy stigma of a strict anabolic steroid. One of the best examples of this is the use of tamoxifen in the treatment of estrogen-receptor-sensitive breast cancer in women. It is currently believed that tamoxifen actively blocks estrogen receptors in the body, and that the resultant anabolic potential may be of either a direct or indirect mechanism. However, some anabolic signs are seen in some women who are taking tamoxifen, such as weight gain and nitrogen retention.

• *women with sexual frigidity*. It is generally accepted that sexual desire in women is highly influenced by the small amount of testosterone in her body under normal conditions. In many cases, sexual frigidity in women may have both psychological and physiological causes, or it may remain a mystery in some women. It has been shown that exogenous testosterone, and probably anabolic steroids may potentiate the orgasmic response in women and greatly influence the libido in some women. Although the level of testosterone in a woman may be a factor in all of the ramifications of sexual desire and sexual interests, it is certainly not the only one. However, it is safe to say that in some women, the use of small quantities of testosterone or other anabolic steroid may be used with dramatic results.

• *women with collagen vascular diseases*. Collagen vascular diseases are a conglomerate of disease states which generally include rheumatoid arthritis, scleroderma and systemic lupus erythematosis, as well as an assortment of other similar arthritic conditions. One of the overriding circumstances in most all of these diseases is that they manifest some type of breakdown in the immune system, more specifically in the aggressiveness of the T-suppressor lymphocytes, which allows the body to destroy itself, especially in the joint regions of the body. These diseases almost always have a considerable state of mental endogenous depression associated with them.

Some early scientific work summarized in *Anabolic Steroids and the Athlete* regarding the use of anabolic steroids in the treatment of these diseases has resulted in some recent renewal of considering these anabolic drugs for this set of diseases. Recently, it has been shown that some men and women have had some major improvements in the disease conditions associated with the collagen vascular disorders by the use of testosterone. The use of the anabolic/androgenic steroids probably boosts the aggressiveness of the T-suppressor lymphocytes and lifts the patient from a state of debilitating mental depression. As with all of the aspects of anabolic steroid therapy in disease states and athletic arenas, this area is in further need of appropriate scientific studies.

• *women with anorexia nervosa.* This condition, which is generally associated with a high mortality rate when full-blown, results in a generalized neuroendocrine-psychological system depression. Anorexia nervosa has become more prominent of late, and it has been considered by some to be a by-product of the "ultra-fitness" syndrome in susceptible women. In its advanced stages, the woman loses most endocrine function and has profound anorexia and aversion to food. And, in the hospitalized patient, the combination of parenteral nutrition techniques combined with low-dose anabolic steroids may prevent the catabolic responses and restore the appetite long enough for the patient to survive and recover. However, at this time, no medical studies have been reported regarding this topic.

Therefore, with the aforementioned presentation as a basis, it can be stated that *in some cases for some women anabolic steroid use has beneficial health effects.*

Athletic Aspects of Anabolic Steroids in Women

Normally, the average woman has approximately 100 times *less* male hormone in her blood serum than does the average man. This tiny amount of male hormone which occurs naturally in women is secreted by the adrenal glands, which are small glands located essentially on the upper aspect of the kidneys. And, since the adrenal glands secrete a variety of hormones and other active molecules, especially in response to stress and exercise, the normal amount of male hormone in normal women may vary to a significant degree. Even in training women athletes, it is this relative lack of male hormone which essentially limits her muscular mass, strength and red blood cell parameters in the blood.

The discussion of anabolic steroid use in women athletes will consist of the following topics:

- beneficial factors on women's athletic performance;

- adverse factors on the health of women athletes;

- special psychological and psychosexual considerations for women athletes.

Before these topics are presented it is important for the reader to accept this point: anabolic steroids and human growth hormone use among women athletes is significant and increasing. Almost every area of sport, and even in some fitness-oriented women who do not compete in any sport, now has women who are using anabolic steroids for their believed beneficial effects on their athletic performance or physique. What serious woman athlete would not wish to add thirty yards or more to her tee shot or add twenty miles per hour to her tennis ground strokes or serves or to reduce her running time in the marathon by several minutes or more? What if she could train with greater intensity and avoid subsequent injuries? Well, the promises of anabolic steroid use for women athletes has several obvious lures such as fame and fortune, but the "hooks" may be in the form of the masculinization of her female body characteristics and a significantly altered psychological profile.

For women athletes, a relatively small amount of exogenous (added) anabolic steroid has *major* effects on her body and her subsequent athletic potentials. This is primarily due to the fact that the woman athlete has, as previously mentioned, a normally tiny amount of male hormone in her body. So, on a percentage-change basis, and for other complex concepts dealing with the balance between the concentrations of "free" hormone and "bound" hormone, a few milligrams of additional daily anabolic steroid for a woman athlete represents a significant change in anabolic potential.

Furthermore, since detection of anabolic steroid use in athletes depends both on the absolute dose taken by the athlete, and the time between taking this dose and the testing time, it is more difficult to detect anabolic steroid use in women athletes by urine testing. In other words, anabolic steroids seem to be effective in enhancing the athletic performance in women athletes in such a low dose that the body's clearing mechanisms reduce the concentrations of the anabolic steroid by-products in the urine below the detectable level rather quickly. Depending on the anabolic steroid selected, a woman athlete could use a regimen of low-dose anabolic steroids up to a few weeks prior to competition and her urine test results would subsequently be "clean." This furthers the interesting dilemma which has created a widening "jealousy gap" among women athletes, and for many women athletes, they are beginning to feel they must resort to the effects of anabolic steroids just to compete, and to worry about any potential adverse conditions later.

Beneficial Factors on Women's Athletic Performance

Since there have been no reported scientific studies on the beneficial effects which anabolic steroids may afford to women athletes, any discussion of this topic must be composed of the following sources of information:

• studies of the effects of anabolic steroids on women with various health disorders which are reported in the medical science literature;

• studies of the effects of anabolic steroids on normal women who are not athletic which are reported in the literature;

• current medical and scientific theories on the subject;

• anecdotal information derived from personal interviews, clinical observations, diary information, longitudinal athletic performance changes and so on.

In order to place credence in anecdotal information, it is imperative to consider something about the persons who have gathered this information. My wife, Susan, has been instrumental in several aspects of this issue, for she has been a registered nurse for over a decade in the medical field of cancer research, and she is knowledgeable about the use of anabolic steroids in these patients. She has completed six marathons and she is an active member of the American Medical Joggers Association. She has been an Official Drug Officer and part of the medical team at the 1984 Women's World Power-lifting Championships in which she helped supervise the International Olympic Committee's (IOC) protocol for the collection and testing of the participants. She has also been active in weight training, she has attended and judged bodybuilding contests for women, and she has attended several national and international sports medicine meetings where experts have discussed anabolic hormone use. Therefore, she has read about, studied, conversed with and urine-tested a variety of women athletes who have discussed some of their concerns about the rising incidence of anabolic hormone use among women athletes. As a result of these aforementioned experiences, and with the hundreds of hours of discussions with me about her anecdotal findings and testimonies, especially regarding the psychological changes in the women athletes using the drugs, her opinions have proved to be invaluable to this topic.

The manner in which anabolic steroid use may afford advantages to a woman's athletic performance stem from both physiological and psychological mechanisms. These are summarized below:

Beneficial Physiological Effects

• increased hemoglobin concentration and increased blood volume which directly enhances maximum aerobic capacity and endurance capacity;

• increased muscle mass formation in response to training which is *over and above* that of athletic training alone;

• tendency to allow for greater reduction in body fat percentage and increases in the lean body mass per pound ratio;

• tendency to cause an increased vascularity to the trained muscles;

• ability to hasten injury healing responses to tendons, muscles and bones, which directly affects the ability to train with greater intensity;

• probable protection against stress fractures;

• reduced post-training period catabolic responses which high-intensity training causes.

Beneficial Psychological Effects

• general "psychological high";

• increased desire to train and excel;

• increased aggressive behavior;

• increased tendency for hostility;

• increased mental intensity and ability to concentrate;

• increased pain tolerance;

• increased inability to accept poor personal performance;

• increased ability to set and achieve goals.

Therefore, with so many potential real avenues to enhance the athletic capacity in women from a strictly beneficial point of view, it is not difficult to understand why anabolic steroid use among women athletes is increasing.

Adverse Factors on the Health of Women Athletes

Any change that a particular drug causes in its user which is not one of the desired effects is usually considered an adverse effect. However, what is a desired effect or a tolerable change for one woman may be quite the opposite for another woman. For instance, anabolic steroids may cause a variety of changes in a woman athlete that have nothing to do with her athletic performance, but for any given woman, some of these changes may or may not be viewed as adverse. However, some of the changes which anabolic steroids can cause

Table 6: Adverse Physical Conditions Occurring in Women Using Anabolic Steroids

Reversible Condition	Partly Reversible	Irreversible
fluid retention	cystic acne	deepening of the voice
hypertension	clitoral enlargement	dark hair on face
"flushed" face	facial pore enlargement	body hair growth
decreased breast size	oily skin	scalp hair loss
non-scarring acne		
menstrual irregularities		

Table 7: Psychological and Behavioral Changes Occurring in Women Using Anabolic Steroids

Factor	On the Drugs	Shortly after Stopping	Ultimate Effects
sex drive	increased	temporary decrease	probable overall increase
sexual pleasure	increased	remains increased	probable overall increase
self-esteem	increased	temporary decrease	probable overall increase
energy level	increased	temporary decrease	probable overall increase
pain tolerance	increased	temporary decrease	probable overall increase
moods	elation	depressive state	reflective self-denial
	aggressiveness	apathy	introspective remorse
	short-tempered	listlessness	
	mental intensity	suicidal thoughts	

primarily in the appearance and psychological make-up of the women who use them would be considered adverse changes by most people.

To further confuse the issue of the adverse conditions associated with anabolic steroid use in women athletes, primarily to the changes in her appearance and psyche, are the following concepts:

• many of the adverse effects are dose-related, time-related, both or neither;

• many of the adverse effects are reversible after the drugs are discontinued, but some of the changes are permanent;

• many of the adverse effects of the drugs occur while the woman is actively taking them;

• some of the adverse effects are seen only after the drugs are discontinued;

• some of the adverse effects seem to have an accumulative nature to them;

• the long-term adverse physical effects on a woman who has used anabolic steriods extensively are not known;

• the long-term adverse *psychological* changes may be the adverse condition of greatest concern.

Tables 6 and 7 (see page 46) contain many of the physically adverse conditions and the psychological and behavioral changes which can occur in a dose-related fashion in women athletes who use anabolic steroids.

Special Psychological and Psychosexual Considerations for Women Athletes Using Anabolic Steroids

Women athletes who use anabolic steroids to enhance their athletic potentials definitely undergo some significant changes in their thought processes, observed psychological profiles, behavioral characteristics, and psychosexual activities. It would be ignorant to really believe that these powerful, essentially male hormone derivatives would not cause psychological changes along with the observed physical changes in women athletes. In fact, there seems to be a much more complex array of disturbances to the natural hormonal balance of women athletes who take anabolic steroids than in the men athletes who take them. These disturbances probably stem from factors revolving around the nature of a primarily estrogen-controlled system converted to a system which may be receiving ambivalent, bipolar or conflicting hormonal imput signals.

In many tissues of the body, the steroid molecules are believed to "compete" for tissue receptors. In other tissues it is currently believed that there are specific receptors for the specific steroid molecules. How these anabolic steroids cause the alterations in mood, thought processes and other obvious psychological changes within the female mind is beyond even the comprehension of the most intuitive experts of our time. But even without an accurate modern theory to explain them, and without any method to scientifically test or prove them, these psychological changes in many women athletes are real, and they may have devastating long-term results.

It has been suggested previously that the hormonal balance of humans is linked in some manner with their thought processes, psychological behavior, and psychosexual behavior. It also seems from clinical observations that exogenous anabolic steroid use in women athletes has a "self-justifying" effect in that the woman's mind is altered in some manner by the influence of these anabolic steroids to accept the resulting body image and appearance changes as a part of herself during the period when she is taking the drugs. This is a very insidious, but extremely important effect which the anabolic steroids cause. However, when the woman athlete discontinues the anabolic steroids, for whatever reasons, there seems to be a progressive internal psychological struggle within herself to accept what she "sees" as herself. In other words, some of the physical changes which tend to be irreversible such as deepening of the voice, acne scars or persistent low-grade acne, and other irreversible ill-defined virilizing facial changes seem to become intolerable to her as the mental influences of the anabolic steroids wear off. This "self-justifying" influence of anabolic steroids is one in which the woman athlete embarking on the use of anabolic steroids to enhance her performance must be educated. Otherwise, in a sense, the woman athlete may eventually become to hate the "monster" which she, or she under the influence of the drugs in the hands of overzealous coaches, trainers, husbands, or boy-friends, has created.

So with the aforementioned discussion, it seems that significant anabolic steroid use by women athletes may result in a long-term psychological unacceptance of herself *and* by society. Once the obvious irreversible changes in appearance occur coupled with the induced psychological alterations, for the woman athlete *there tends to be no return to the pre-steroid state*. In other words, anabolic steroid use tends to be a one-way street for the woman athlete. It is very difficult for the woman athlete with a bass-like voice, significant facial hair, acne, a virilized face, a highly muscular physique, and complex psychological alterations to currently fit into the flow of society. These changes in the woman may prove to be a tragedy beyond the scope of the simple definition of a "side effect."

Since the definition of adulthood in the United States is an arbitrary one and is generally one assigned to the later teenage years, most adults here have the privilege to determine which of the many avenues of life they will take. In consequence, many young adult athletes will tend to choose some directions prior to becoming fully educated in the route they are selecting, and thus we must continue to thrust forward with their education. In most cases, an ounce of edu-cation is worth at least a pound of cure.

Although the potential benefits which anabolic steroids afford to athletic performance have not been fully elucidated, they cannot be denied. But, for every athletic champion which anabolic steroids help to create, there will be many non-champion anabolic steroid-using athletes who will eventually attest to the significant physical and mental ailments induced by these drugs.

It is likely safe to say that there are some of the less androgenic anabolic steroids which some women athletes could take at low doses and avoid many of the virilizing effects. However, there are no studies to support this concept. Currently, it seems that the competitive woman athlete who must face urine drug testing measures is turning to the use of testosterone itself instead of the synthetic less-virilizing anabolic steroids. This is due to the fact that it is more difficult to accurately detect the use of testosterone, for even with the newly implemented test for testosterone, its detection relies on a partially subjective ratio measurement. This ratio measurement is based on the normal ratio in the urine of testosterone and epitestosterone (an epimer metabolite of testosterone) and is one to one. Therefore, it is proposed that any additional testosterone which the athlete takes will upset this balance, which can now be measured in the urine. It is difficult to determine how much confidence to place in this test, and for the 1984 Olympic Games, a ratio of six to one was the cut-off ratio. This means that an athlete can still use limited amounts of testosterone, even just prior to and during the Games and "pass" the urine test. So, in effect, urine testing in women has forced the women using the less virilizing anabolic steroids to now use the more virilizing testosterone! But, to circumvent this entire situation, many experts, including Olympic coaches and trainers, agree that the men and women athletes are using human growth hormone, and that the incidence is increasing.

Summary

In this part several aspects of anabolic steroid use by women have been presented. And, as provided in the introduction to this part, I would again prefer to select some important quotes from the famous science fiction author H.G. Wells taken from *The Mind at the End of Its Tether*.

> The philosophical mind is not what people would call a healthy buoyant mind. That 'healthy mind' takes life as it finds it and troubles no more about that. None of us start life as philosophers. We become philosophers sooner or later, or we die before we become philosophical. The realization of limitation and frustration is the beginning of the bitter wisdom of philosophy, and of this, that 'healthy mind,' by its innate gift for incoherence and piecemeal evasion and credulity, never knows. Mind may be near the end of its tether, and yet that everyday drama will go on because it is the normal make-up of life and there is nothing else to replace it.

Many readers of this text will not be able to distinguish the subtle differences between opinions, emotions, and philosophies. In any controversial issue, these differences, although they seem the same, provide the basis for solutions. Opinions usually lack the facts, and emotions tend to override the more factual opinions. However, as stated above, a philosophical approach is attained only after the passage of time has allowed for the philosopher to reflect and dwell on an issue from many perspectives.

My personal philosophy regarding the use of anabolic steroids by women athletes is one of remorseful cynicism. I am not sure that anything which I say or do will alter this horrible evolutionary direction for which athletic womanhood is headed. In effect, what is happening is that American athletes are allowing the irrational morals of other powerful countries to influence our young people; and all under the auspices of internationally acclaimed athletic success which is then converted to major promotional forces for nationalism during cold war times. And in this way, women athletes who alter their bodies and minds by anabolic hormones, and who subsequently win on an international basis, are nothing more than governmental instruments. But, the saddest result of this approach lies with the overwhelming numbers of athletic young women who will sacrifice many of the finer qualities of womanhood for nothing and will have no method of recuperation.

In his last in a long line of books, H.G. Wells, at the age of 79 years wrote:

> The writer sees the world as a jaded world devoid of recuperative power. In the past he has liked to think that Man could pull out of his entanglements and start a new creative phase of human living. In the face of our universal inadequacy, that optimism has given place to a stoical cynicism. The old men behave for the most part meanly and disgustingly, and the young are spasmodic, foolish and all too easily misled. Man must go steeply up or down and the odds seem to be all in favour of his going down and out. If he goes up, then so great is the adaptation demanded of him that he must cease to be a man. Ordinary man is at the end of his tether.
>
> It is possible that there are wide variations in the mental adaptability of contemporary mankind. It is possible that the mass of contemporary mankind may not be as readily accessible to fresh ideas as the younger, more childish minds of earlier generations, and it is also possible that hard imaginative thinking has not increased so as to keep pace with the expansion and complication of human societies and organizations. That is the darkest shadow upon the hopes of mankind.

3

Human Growth Hormone and Gigantism

As our minds have probed more and more curiously into the space-time continuum in which the drama of evolution has been framed, they have discovered one paradoxical aspect after another behind the plausible face of "normal" being.... In the record of the rocks it is always the gigantic individuals who appear at the end of each chapter.

H.G. Wells,
The Mind at the End of Its Tether (1946)

Introduction

In the previous parts of this book, many of the aspects involving the athletic uses of anabolic steroids were presented. The various parameters of this issue have developed over the past fifteen years and they have intensified recently. Indeed, the anabolic steroid issue is now an international dilemma that persists in spite of national and international medical and sports medicine meetings designed to discuss the topic. Basically, these attempts have failed because, for the most part, the issue probably has no simple solution. Some of the reasons for the continuing dilemma center on various aspects of medical ethics, the philosophical aspects of winning, the problems in defining athletic worth, the previous unforgivable untruths promoted by

current method exists for distinguishing whether or not an athlete is using the hormone, due primarily to the following reasons:

(1) Pituitary extract human growth hormone and the synthetic versions of human growth hormone are nearly indistinguishable from the naturally produced hormone by current testing equipment.

(2) The half-life of human growth hormone is so short, that the hormone would be out of the body before current athletic testing procedures could detect it.

In other words, an injection of human growth hormone would be undetectable within a few hours of the injection time, even if there were a test for it. This happens because human growth hormone sets up a cascade of events, some of which are carried out by the "messenger molecules," which cause the contructive effects on human metabolism, and then the human growth hormone itself is quickly removed from the body.

In addition, there seems to be few viable ideas regarding future methods for detecting athletes who use this hormone for enhancing athletic skills, or for future children who may be injected with this hormone for subsequent athletic enhancement and height gains. However, there may be some remote idea possibilities based on the following rationale:

(1) The new synthetic versions could possibly be formulated with some different amino acids in various positions on the current amino acid sequence. This would make the synthetic versions analogs of the true human growth hormone molecules, and possibly make them detectable without destroying the activity of the hormone. It is known that the amino acid sequence directly affects the tertiary molecular structure, but not all of the amino acids in "non-key" positions need be identical to those in the natural hormone. So, it may be possible to introduce differing amino acids at various points in the molecular sequence and not affect the resulting tertiary structure enough to change its subsequent activity appreciably. And, in many cases when analogs of other hormones are synthesized, the analog is more potent than the natural hormone for certain functions. However,

this approach to detecting athletic use of human growth hormone would be expensive, for the scientists would have to go back to the initial steps of instructing the bacteria to now place different amino acids into the hormone molecule. But this could be a viable solution to the widespread misuse of human growth hormone, especially in athletics.

(2) The antibody formation to chronic injections of human growth hormone in some cases could provide medical scientists with some newer approaches to direct the drug testing equipment. However, at this time no good ideas have been promoted along these lines, and if a method becomes available, the costs to employ it may be prohibitive for the sporting institutions.

So, even with these and possibly other ideas to render human growth hormone use by athletes detectable, it is safe to say that it is untraceable at this time.

The previous discussion has helped to serve the following concept: that the misuse of human growth hormone may produce human athletic giants, and its misuse is likely to become widespread as more human growth hormone is mass-produced, and that the scope in solving this predicament does not lie in simple drug testing procedures. This discussion has also ushered in the concept of "selective gigantism." And, although the misuse of human growth hormone may result in this form of iatrogenic giants, it may not be the only synthetic anabolic hormone springing from the vats of genetically engineered bacteria with this capability. Therefore, this introduction of "selective gigantism" should be carried through the remainder of this book as a theme.

Selective gigantism simply refers to the selection of persons to become structural giants via anabolic hormonal manipulation. Choosing the proper hormones for this monstrous undertaking is part of the process, and so are the people who will ultimately do the selecting. Who will choose the children to be inflicted with this bizarre method of hormonal manipulation? Will the minor child decide? Or will it be the parents of the child, or perhaps a group of sporting officials under the auspices of governmental nationalism? Others to consider would be wealthy sports sponsors. But in this burgeoning era of "liability law," will it be the government who selects the children, maybe even children of yours? And, if not in this country, how about in the countries where human rights are engulfed in the sea of de-humanization? And, if the Soviets practice the ludicrous art of "selective gigantism" to beat our American athletes, will we begrudgingly follow their lead and allow our children to be "nationalistic pawns" to promote athletics, winning, and the democratic style of life? Indeed, these are heavy questions to answer. In my opinion, it is doubtful that anyone will be able to accept the liability of "selective gigantism."

There comes a point in many athletes' adolescence where height becomes somewhat of a limiting factor in athletic performance and future athletic career opportunities. Those of us who have been involved with athletics as children and adolescents can easily relate to just how important it seems to be just a few inches taller. And, indeed, in many sports, a few inches of additional height is usually beneficial to the athlete, and it may afford the difference between stardom and mediocrity. Furthermore, this difference between stardom and mediocrity may be readily converted to a financial fortune for select "superstars." If most children are left to decide whether they wish to be taller or not, the usual response would favor the increased stature.

There is no doubt as to the motivating forces of peer pressure. And for the young, striving athlete, the question of whether or not to use athletic enhancing drugs is part of this peer pressure. And, if peer pressure has its way, it is either take the anabolic hormones or don't play. Unfortunately, this is becoming a more difficult decision for the young athlete to make. So, from the child turned young athlete's point of view, "selective gigantism" may become a real phenomenon.

Usually, parents of athletic children who may have a bright future in athletics possess mixed feelings about anabolic hormone use in their children. However, even the most persuasive parents have some evident internal strifes which they must answer to regarding the concept of hormonal manipulation of the athletic children. This can be detected in the letter (see page 68) which was sent to me in September 1983.

As the parent in this letter indicated, he can see "no cons with making him taller." However, there may be disadvantages to such a program of "selective gigantism." If the overproduction and probable overuse of human growth hormone continues into adult life, it may be responsible for a group of abnormalities known as *acromegaly*. The major features of acromegaly include bony overgrowths in the skull and in other bones, soft tissue overgrowths, thickening of the skin, diabetes mellitus, cardiovascular disease, goiters, menstrual disorders,

Dear Dr. Taylor:

Thank you for your time talking to me about human growth hormone. I know that you must have received hundreds of calls regarding this issue.

My son is 15 years old and stands 5'6". He plays quarterback in football, plays shortstop in baseball, wrestles and is a good all-around athlete. I don't know if he has aspirations for professional athletics; however, he is very conscious of his height. Since I'm only 5'6" and his mother is only 5'0", he has probably already reached his height.

I hope everything works out for you. I know that making decisions such as these must place you under a lot of pressure. I travel all over the country and would like my son to talk to you. After all, it is his life and I want him to make any decisions about his future. All that I can do is to provide him with the pros and cons (although I cannot find any cons with making him taller) and help him as much as I can. I will pay you anything you ask for this help. I look forward to reading your book, *Anabolic Steroids and the Athlete*, and I would like to read any material which you have compiled on human growth hormone and athletics.

I enjoyed talking with your wife, Susan on the phone. I know that she must be going through most of this with you.

Best of Luck,
BC

decreased sexual desire and impotence. Acromegaly almost always shortens the life span of the persons it afflicts.

In clinical terms, the group of bodily characteristics describing acromegaly was first used in the late 1880's. Since that time the acromegaly syndrome has been studied by several research groups in an attempt to define the physical and clinical changes associated with the syndrome. *Acromegaly* is composed of two Greek roots: "acr-" and "megal." *Acr-* relates to the peripheral body parts such as the arms, legs, hands, fingers, toes, nose and so on. *Megal-* means large. Therefore, as simplistic initial attempts to describe this phenomenon were made, the clinical observations of enlarged fingers, ears, nose and toes became the hallmark of the characteristic body changes.

As autopsies become a more popular method for correlating the pathophysiology occurring within the person afflicted with this syndrome, it was found that many, if not most, of the acromegalic patients had enlarged pituitary glands or actual tumors in the anterior pituitary gland. These tumors indeed had functional capacity to over-produce human growth hormone through various mechanisms of stimulation, and today, it is well-documented that the acromegaly syndrome is caused by a chronic overproduction of human growth hormone or from a chronically overactive growth hormone axis. The main clinical findings of the acromegaly syndrome are contained in Table 8 (see page 70).

Without discussing each of these major clinical conditions, it is important to understand some of the other general aspects of the acromegaly syndrome. These general aspects listed below are:

• Acromegaly usually becomes obvious in the third or fourth decade of life in persons who have had chronic overstimulation of the growth hormone axis. These changes are largely irreversible once they occur. In general, as seen in nature, the acromegaly syndrome is observed after several years of over-production of growth hormone;

• Acromegaly usually has afflicted men and women on an equal basis.

• The acromegaly syndrome usually shortens an afflicted person's life span by approximately 20 years or more.

• The classic acromegalic appearance is comprised of "drumstick" fingers and toes, "spade-like" hands with a ring size of "20" or more, very large ears and a very large nose, changes in the jawbone size resulting in large gaps between the bottom teeth and a severe "overbite," frontal bossing (overgrowth of the skull and soft tissues above the eyes), and abnormal bone and soft tissue growth in the areas where muscle tendons attach to the bones.

A new generation of acromegalics may occur subsequent to the chronic use of various growth hormone releasing agents, such as amino acid preparations, or by chronic injections of human growth hormone or primate growth hormone by athletes. Furthermore, another future generation of *athletic acromegalics* may occur if the somatomedins, growth factors and multiplication factors are also manufactured via recombinant-DNA genetic engineering techniques. Anecdotal reports of adult athletes with acromegalic signs resulting from the injections of human growth hormone and primate growth hormone have already been reported in athletic circles.

Table 8: Main Clinical Characteristics of the Acromegaly Syndrome

Condition	Davidoff (1926)	Gordon (1962)	Lawrence (1970)	Hofeldt (1973)	Tyrrell (1978)	Klijn (1980)	Jadresic (1982)
Acral enlargment with soft tissue overgrowth	100%	100%	98%	96%	100%	100%	100%
Diabetes mellitus	25%	47%	38%	60%	50%	30%	27%
Cardiac disorders	–	–	–	12%	16%	23%	34%
Goiter	25%	24%	–	18%	32%	41%	27%
Decreased libido & impotence	38%	27%	40%	27%	46%	43%	40%
Menstrual disorders in women	87%	63%	80%	32%	60%	52%	77%
Hypertension	–	18%	–	23%	24%	20%	34%
Hyperhydrosis (excess sweating)	60%	–	80%	88%	88%	82%	65%

Will the Use of hGH in Athletes Cause Acromegaly?

For any athlete who uses human growth hormone or primate growth hormone on a regular basis, the concurrent development or future development of the acromegaly syndrome is a real threat. And, if any athlete examines the clinical conditions which are part of being an acromegalic athlete, especially if the signs and changes occur by thirty years of age or so, then the athlete will realize that chronic growth hormone use indeed is risky to his/her health. In my opinion, excessive production of, injection of, or artificial stimulatory release of human growth hormone will cause the acromegaly syndrome in a time-related, dose-related fashion in some athletes.

However, a single injection of hGH will not cause acromegaly in any athlete, and neither will several injections of the hormone. But as the injections continue, probably even with cyclical periods of injections, many athletes will develop the acromegaly syndrome and die prematurely. Again, this will be a function of the actual total amount of human growth hormone injected or excessively released and the actual duration of the injections. In this manner then, by the time the athlete has chronically injected human growth hormone into his/her body, it may be too late to reverse the acromegalic changes which have occurred or that will occur. Although it is difficult for a physician to assess the "worth" of this type of hormonal manipulation for an athlete who is self-administering the hormone, it is easy for me to declare the potential risks involved; the risks are as glaring as in the first patient which I examined with acromegaly! His hands and fingers were huge, and the ends of his fingers were larger than at their bases. He was so weak with diabetes that he was bedridden. His muscles were wasted and his skin was very thick, especially on the soles of his feet, and he had little or no sensation in this thick skin. When he smiled, his teeth appeared to be ½-inch apart. His nose was that of a cauliflower, and a large stalk at that. His ears were thrice the normal size and malformed due to the excessive growth which had occurred. When I listened to his heart, I really did not need a stethoscope, for his heart made such abnormal noises that they could be heard over a foot away. He claimed not to have had an erection in many years and talking about this subject made him very unhappy. I'll never forget how sad I was when I learned that he was only 44 years old, for he appeared to be at least 65 years of age! Without a doubt, this man was not a picture of strength and health, and he was assigned to my medical service when I was a student.

As I taught this man to inject his daily insulin, I wondered what had made this man wait so long before seeking medical help. His skin was so thick and tough that a needle would pass it only with unusual force. He claimed that the changes were gradual over a few years, and it was his lack of sexual function that made his wife finally realize that this syndrome would not go away. By the time this man had sought medical attention, his diabetes was severe and he subsequently died in the hospital with pneumonia due to his inability to fight off an otherwise simple infection.

With drastically more human growth hormone available, with the well-established black market distribution network already awaiting the claimed abundance of hGH, and with the nearly insatiable desire for some athletes to use this powerful hormone, *athletic acromegaly* will probably become a new medical syndrome in the 1990's. As with anabolic steroid use, athletes are currently using much larger doses than they did just five years ago; and in many cases the quantities used are over an order of magnitude greater. So, if this athletic version of "the blind leading the blind" logic is transferred to the self-experimental use of human growth hormone, then athletic acromegaly will become a reality rather quickly.

Prior to the promised abundance of human growth hormone, medical scientists have actually been unable to determine what the optimum replacement doses are for dwarf children. And, some scientists feel that with the increased supply of the hormone, the optimum doses found may be significantly greater than what is currently used to treat these children. A few medical studies have indicated that the response to human growth hormone injections is dose-related to a degree, but how far this dose-response factor extends to enhancing the growth of otherwise normal children is surely unknown at this time. Athletes, as well, have probably used suboptimal doses due to this shortage situation. Will signs of the athletic acromegaly syndrome serve as an end point of what is more than optimal human growth hormone? If not, what parameters will the medical scientists use to determine what is optimal human growth hormone use? Hopefully, it will be an adverse condition which is reversible, for the changes seen with acromegaly are irreversible ones.

An interesting phenomenon is forming in the United States and some other modern countries across the globe known as the "reverse pyramid" with regard to the numbers of aged persons compared to the number of present and future young persons. In all previous times, the age distribution of humanity resembled a pyramid, with the widest base of people being young, and with the tip of the pyramid representing the small numbers of older persons. However, this situation is changing rather rapidly on an ecological time frame, and the concept of the "reverse pyramid" is predicted by some scientists to become a reality as early as the mid-21st century.

For the sake of an educated hypothetical situation, let us combine the concepts of "selective gigantism" via hormone-induced persons with the concept of the "reverse pyramid." Furthermore, let us speculate that, for a variety of sound and unsound reasons, "selective gigantism" and hormonal manipulation of young persons in the very near future becomes widespread. Then, if these hormonally manipulated people live into the 21st century, then a large portion of the older persons who make up the top portion of the "reverse pyramid" will be products of hormonal manipulation, and may be the norm for humanity. Then, if humanity is destroyed in any of a number of currently speculated ways, then the science fiction writings of H.G. Wells which were presented at the beginning of this part would then become profoundly predictive. Indeed, then "In the record of the rocks [fossils] it is always the gigantic individuals who appear at the end of each chapter."

Discussion and Summary

Everyone knows that sports sponsorship can be very lucrative, especially in recent times. In the remaining years of the 20th century, the successful sports entrepreneur just might take a place in history and literature analagous to that of the great industrial and banking entrepreneurs of the 19th century.

In 1977 novelist Peter Lear depicted some of the current and moral questions of modern athletics and of modern society in his book *Goldengirl*. Portrayed is a web of character flaws and plot complications coupled with real-life "selective gigantism" medications such as anabolic steroids and human growth hormone. Lear warns us through the power of his pen that humans *use* other humans for their own ends—in this case for those two familiar roots of evil: money and power. Lear shows how the genius of a medical scientist, the compulsiveness of a coach (an erstwhile "Olympic hopeful"), the persuasive powers of a sports psychologist, the greed of a pharmacist, the ego of a wealthy sports sponsor and the genetic potential of an athletic young girl all combine to create a monstrous victim called Goldengirl.

These assorted adults "program" the girl to win three Olympic gold medals at the 1980 Moscow Olympic Games. In the story, Goldengirl does not know that she is actually the product of anabolic hormonal manipulation until she develops a severe case of diabetes from the chronic human growth hormone injections. This event forces the medical scientist, her father, to confess his experiment publicly. Lear depicts the medical scientist as having been driven to publish his theories on human growth and development in the scientific literature to make the potential properties and abuse of anabolic steroids and human growth hormone a "truth, secure for the rest of time." The medical scientist did so, as the reader learns, by using his own daughter for the experiment. Furthermore, the adverse effects of these anabolic hormones altered Goldengirl's normal feminine facial appearance and physique so drastically that she had to undergo multiple plastic surgery procedures so that she would be subsequently acceptable as a woman athletic champion by the American public. Also, Goldengirl was under continuous psychotherapy by a sports psychologist, and this need most probably was due to the girl's un-acceptance of herself and her grossly underdeveloped social self.

Goldengirl has value because it shows the operation of the human conscience, which is a marvelous and truly divine character-istic. Lear shows that eventually everyone must answer to conscience despite our tremendous ability to rationalize our responses to events and ideas. The medical scientist in Lear's book satisfactorily proves his theory on human growth and development via "selective gigan-tism" techniques, but in doing so he goes beyond his ability to rationa-lize away the truth of what he had done to his daughter. After he is forced to disclose to his daughter, Goldengirl, his role in the experi-ment, she rejects and curses him. Subsequently, the medical scientist cannot cope with this turn of events and he becomes irrational and commits suicide!

Alfred Nobel discovered dynamite and hoped that his dis-covery would be of benefit to mankind. Perhaps dynamite has helped some people, but it also has been responsible for much human suffering and death. Because he lived to see the horrible misuse of his genius, the remorseful Nobel provided that the money from his estate be awarded to deserving individuals in the fields of medicine, peace and related scientific fields. Nobel's actions may also be exemplified by a concept credited to the 18th century English poet, William Blake. Mr. Blake never heard of anabolic hormones or "selective gigantism" or of the potential risks involved with the hormonal manipulation of athletes, but in many ways, a statement attributed to him may shed some light on this important issue: "You never know what is enough, unless you know what is more than enough!"

By the time we indeed determine what is more than enough added synthetic human growth hormone, it may be too late to reduce or cope with the human suffering which such misuse will cause. Much potential for destruction exists in the widespread misuse of human growth hormone for seemingly good intentions. Therefore, we must not allow this type of "dynamite" to backfire on humanity! Admittedly, this is an idealistic notion. Perhaps it is more realistic to expect that the promises of power, huge profits, and athletic success resulting from hormonal tampering will cause an explosion of exploitation and human suffering which may be impossible to halt.

Twenty-five years ago, a novel laboratory method was developed for creating polypeptide molecules by Dr. R. Bruce Merrifield. And, subsequent to the use of his unusual development, known as the "Merrifield Methodology," he was the only U.S. scientist awarded a Nobel Prize in 1984. According to the Royal Swedish Academy of Sciences, "Merrifield's Methodology" has brought about a revolution in peptide and protein chemistry, and thousands of peptides and polypetides have now been synthesized using this approach. Scientists working on nucleic acids, rather than polypeptides, have also benefited from the "Merrifield Method." Some automated apparatuses, sometimes referred to as "gene machines," are programmed to synthesize chains of nucleic acids. These nucleotide chains are an all important tool used in genetic engineering. There is no question that this discovery has greatly stimulated progress in biochemistry, molecular biology, pharmacology, and medicine. But, what is of unknown concern, is whether discoveries such as these are collectively beneficial to mankind. Therefore, keeping the intent of the Nobel Prize in mind, it becomes evident that the *use* and *control* of outstanding inventions is just as important as the discovery itself.

On the basis of all of the aforementioned concepts and facts, I have consistently suggested that the U.S. Food and Drug Administration reclassify synthetic human growth hormone as a highly controlled drug. If you care about the health of the upcoming athletes, then you must agree. If not, then the next few parts may convince you that all of the synthetic anabolic hormones should be controlled drugs.

This recommendation can be further expanded to include the following suggestions to minimize the traumatic terrors associated with the future widespread misuse of human growth hormone:

(1) classification of all synthetic human growth hormones and analogs by the FDA as highly controlled drugs so that every vial's whereabouts is known, documented, and accounted for by a medical professional;

(2) experimentation allowed in approved laboratories only, and only by expert endocrinologists to determine the safety and effectiveness of the hormone in the closely-related field of pediatric endocrinology;

(3) as further medical indications for human growth hormone are defined and studied in the aforementioned laboratories, then allow the hormone to be prescribed as a schedule II drug with a specific diagnosis accompanying each prescription;

(4) as even further medical indications for human growth hormone expand, the initial highly controlled status of the hormone should be reevaluated for reduced control by the FDA; and

(5) until such time as there is an indication for "general" prescription use by physicians, it makes absolutely no sense to allow human growth hormone to be placed in the general prescription category for this will allow for an immediate abuse situation.

Currently, the country's major medical lawmakers are at odds regarding the release of synthetic human growth hormone. This situation stems from severe clashes over the rights and freedoms of the involved Americans, and ultimately, for people of other nations. Through seemingly helpful intentions and human genius obtained after years of scientific dedication, medical scientists have introduced a method from mass-producing another of the body's powerful hormones. The controlled use of synthetic human growth hormone is just as important as the scientific work devised to identify, isolate, and synthesize it. Once the release of this synthetic human growth hormone away from strict medical science settings and into the control of private enterprises occurs, it may be impossible to recover from the potential abuses of the hormone. However, with the private sector pushing for its release, the nation's medical lawmakers must make their decisions on the human growth hormone issue prior to knowing all of the facts. Furthermore, it is not simply a human growth hormone issue, for in the near future other anabolic hormones will certainly have to be judged by the FDA. Some of these other anabolic hormones will be discussed in the later parts of this book.

4

Using an Organ to Alter Itself: Growth Hormone Releasing Hormones

The postwar period ushered in a new era of biologic research, spurred by the discovery of antibiotics. Suddenly there was both enthusiasm and money for biology, and a torrent of discoveries poured forth: tranquilizers, steroid hormones, immunochemistry, the genetic code. By 1953 the first kidney was transplanted and by 1958 the first birth-control pills were tested. It was not long before biology was the fastest-growing field in all science; it was doubling its knowledge every ten years. Farsighted researchers talked seriously of changing genes, controlling evolution, regulating the mind—ideas that had been wild speculation ten years before. And yet there had never been a biologic crisis.... A crisis is made by men, who enter into the crisis with their own prejudices, propensities, and predispositions. A crisis is the sum of intuition and blind spots, a blend of facts noted and facts ignored. Yet underlying the uniqueness of each crisis is a disturbing sameness. A characteristic of all crises is their predictability, in retrospect. They seem to have a certain inevitability, they seem predestined. This is not true of all crises, but it is true of sufficiently many to make the most hardened historian cynical and misanthropic.

Michael Crichton,
The Andromeda Strain (1969)

Introduction

After reading the first three parts of this book dealing with the issues of the variety of performance — enhancing anabolic hormones used by modern athletes, the reader should become more aware of the scope and seriousness of this phenomenon. It has expanded to become an interdisciplinary, intergenerational, and international dilemma. In other words, this situation has engulfed athletes and children who will become athletes, the coaches, trainers, and parents of these athletes, medical physicians, sporting officials and government officials.

Simply put, present and future athletic excellence is a function of the following parameters:

- having superb genetic endowment for the selected sport;

- utilizing sound training techniques for the selected sport;

- utilizing sound nutritional habits and supplementation;

- receiving appropriate medical/surgical treatment for injuries;

- receiving appropriate psychological and sport-specific strategic support therapy;

- having the ability to obtain mental and physical peaking-effects at contest times;

- having the ability to avoid major injury and to incorporate specific personal trial-and-error learned attributes and scientific knowledge to aid performance;

- having the ability to incorporate ergogenic drugs, such as anabolic steroids and other anabolic hormones into the complex mesh of the above parameters;

- having the ability to use "banned" drugs, as for the Olympic Games, and utilize methods to avoid a "positive" urine test;

• having the ability to alter genetic expression and genetic endowment for maximizing athletic potential via use of growth hormone and other growth enhancing hormones.

The majority of the experts who are knowledgeable of these parameters and their effects on athletic performance are begrudgingly beginning to accept the importance of the anabolic hormone use by athletes in many sports. Also, most athletes would really prefer *not* to have to use these anabolic hormones and other ergogenic drugs for now these drugs have become almost a "necessary evil" to the athletes who are achieving athletic excellence.

On an international basis there seem to be two different, highly successful strategies used in the training of young athletes for eventual athletic competition at international levels. These two methods of "programming" athletic success will be discussed below.

Early Recruitment and Support Approach

Some of the countries of the Eastern Bloc select children at about age ten years or so in terms of their genetic endowment to become future athletes. Then, for approximately two years, these selected children are observed to determine which areas of sport they would most likely excel in based on these two years or so of observation and their genetic make-up. So, at approximately age 12, their training begins, sometimes at the expense of family ties, especially when the children are removed from their families to train.

After this phase of early recruitment, the support phase is incorporated into these athletic children. Their progress is monitored closely and strict training schedules are adhered to, usually in the presence of their coaches and medical doctors. Therefore, in this manner, the Eastern Bloc countries have been able to select the most genetically endowed children to be monitored and taught to be successful athletes. The incentive for the athletic child to excel lies in his/her being able to attain a better position in life within their country and to represent his/her country through athletic achievement. Of course, this type of close support throughout the growth and development phases of late childhood and early adolescence lends itself to hormonal manipulation, especially when the leadership of the country selects and supports the athletic child toward further national cohesiveness and international standing.

No country wishes to admit that its athletes have been hormonally manipulated in order to improve their athletic performances, for it is the "Super Race" idea of genetic excellence that the entire concept of international athletic competition breeds. In other words, all countries seem to wish to credit winning athletes based on which country they live in and how hard they trained and not to factors like anabolic hormones. It is difficult for a particular country to "brag" about the amount of anabolic hormones their athletes have to take to win medals!

As a corollary, no one in the horse racing arena wishes to admit to any hormonal manipulation of their horses, because as an end-product, the promotion that genetics is the overwhelming factor for successful winning horses keeps the stud fees of selected horses at a premium of over $40,000 per stud service. If it got out that some horses could win some major horse racing events due to the influences of anabolic hormones or other drugs, which ultimately were not detected by current postracing testing methods, then how much longer could the horse race promotors continue to retain $40,000 for a stud service? What if a given above-average horse could win due to hypertransfusion of red blood cells a week or so prior to a given race? This particular technique, which is not detectable in elite human athletes and has been shown to significantly reduce running times in as little as three miles races for men, is probably directly transferable to horse racing. If so, then, the concept that genetics is the prime factor in winning would no longer be applicable.

Early Competition and Financial Reward Approach

In the United States most of our internationally competitive athletes have survived rather lengthy bouts of "survival of the fittest." The majority of young citizens have a chance at athletic success and athletic careers, but this chance must usually withstand the challenges of fellow athletes. Although sports medicine, nutrition, and training techniques have made great strides in this country in assisting athletes, sports sponsorship monies from direct and indirect sources have given many athletes the needed extra motivation factor. During the past decade, the number of hours of commercial and cable television coverage of sporting events has increased over two orders of magnitude. Professional athletic contracts have continued to skyrocket in both numbers and in remuneration value. Popular sporting figures through this expanded media coverage have become the "Cold War" idols for many Americans.

The United States has continued to propagate much of its international athletic success due to the extremely broad base of genetic potential within the people who live in the country. This broad base of genetic endowment essentially has come from the influx and interbreeding of the many racial and ethnic backgrounds which coexist within its borders. And, by progressively holding a larger and larger dollar sign in front of our young athletes, the United States has continued to achieve substantial athletic success internationally. However, the United States has continually tried to down play this advantage of its broad-based genetic pool, and instead it has continued to claim that it is the democratic style of life which has been the dominant factor for its international athletic success.

As it stands currently, the concept of hormonal manipulation of athletes is inconsistent with either the genetic quality promotion or the free-world democratic life-style promotion for athletic excellence. It does, however, fit nicely into the ever-luring force of the incredible contracts and support monies offered to reward American and foreign athletic success. Hormonal manipulation of athletes and financial manipulation of athletes may well go hand-in-hand.

Another area in which hormonal manipulation of athletes is currently taking place will now be presented. This area involves the use of growth hormone releasing agents and stimuli to augment human growth hormone releasing patterns.

According to the currently acceptable principles of endocrinology, the following schematic may be constructed in order to define the interrelationships among the growth hormone releasers, human growth hormone, somatomedins, growth factors, and multiplication factors. From this basic schematic it can be demonstrated that, at the hypothalamic level, the positive stimuli cause a release of growth hormone releasing hormone, GHRH, a small peptide hormone. This GHRH is released into a specialized area of the bloodstream which tends to flow directly to the pituitary gland, and GHRH thus stimulates the pituitary gland to release human growth hormone into the generalized bloodstream. Ultimately, this growth hormone release

Figure 2: Schematic of Growth Hormone Release

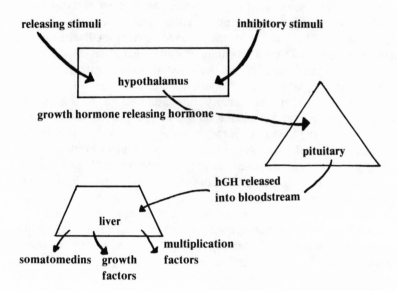

(From Taylor, *Anabolic Steroids*, 1982)

stimulates the liver to produce a variety of small polypeptide molecules known as somatomedins, growth factors, and multiplication factors. These molecules are believed to control many facets of human growth and development more specifically than human growth hormone does.

Therefore, it can be shown that, in this complex pathway which is the major pathway for controlling human growth, there are several points in which exogenous stimuli, drugs, or other hormones may *drive* the system to augment human growth and development.

Physiological Growth Hormone Releasers

The areas of research with growth hormone releasing agents and the conditions which cause growth hormone release exist primarily due to the efforts involved with enabling physicians to determine whether or not a "slow-growing" child has an adequate growth hormone release to provocative stimuli. This has evolved even further to allow medical scientists to gain further knowledge regarding the specific factors which control and regulate human growth and development. But, knowledge in one selected area of medical research sometimes alters in a significant manner some other areas of science or of basic life. This seems to be the case with the entire metabolic growth hormone pathway and modern athletics.

Currently, there are nearly one hundred medical research groups conducting further studies on the various control mechanisms associated with the human growth hormone pathway. Unlike most of the other hormonal pathways in the body, the control mechanism of human growth hormone release is not an end-product negative feedback mechanism. The metabolic control of human growth hormone release is probably the most complex hormonal system in the human body. So many physiological conditions and other stimuli, along with specific drugs, alter human growth hormone release that there is no wonder that we are all of differing heights. Normal adults can range from 4½ feet in height to over 7½ feet.

In a simplistic manner, it is easily claimed and promoted, and then forgotten, that a person's height is genetically determined. This is probably false. More accurately, what *is* genetically determined is the manner in which growth hormone release is responsive to various physiological stimuli, and latently, through various drugs and metabolites which may stimulate the hypothalamus to release GHRH. Also, since there are many known conditions, metabolites, and drugs which can inhibit at the hypothalamic level the release of growth hormone, then what is probably genetically determined is a multifactoral array including:

• the degree of hypothalamic sensitivity to environmental, physiological, metabolic and drug-induced conditions;

• the degree of sensitivity which the pituitary gland has for the previously released GHRH and its subsequent release of growth hormone;

• the degree of sensitivity which the liver possesses for released growth hormone or exogenous growth hormone and its subsequent release of the somatomedins, growth factors and multiplication factors;

• the degree of sensitivity which the tissues possess for the released somatomedins, growth factors, and multiplication factors.

Until recently, the height which a particular person ultimately attained was determined by this genetic dominance alone. Recent studies have begun to show some interesting phenomena in regard to the increasing adult height in the United States. Apparently, children in the United States have some unique characteristics associated with their growth and development years:

(1) The average age of the onset of puberty, especially in young girls, is decreasing for each consecutive generation.

(2) The average number of years which the American child spends in puberty is increasing slightly, and this period of time for the American child is longer than most other countries already.

(3) The quantities of red meat products and meat in general consumed by the American child is higher than other countries.

(4) The quantities of stress or perceived stress associated with growing from childhood to adulthood in the United States are alarming and increasing.

As a result of these aforementioned facts and perhaps some others, the average height of American adults continues to rise significantly every generation. And, essentially, one must wonder if this phenomenon is a product of a genetic change or of changes which are altering the genetic expression of height. As will be discussed later in this part, there are factors between the lines of the above facts which may be altering growth hormone release in our children. Given the longer puberty period for which subtle and some not so subtle changes in growth hormone release to act upon, it is safe to say that some changes in growth hormone release patterns are probably taking place through changes in environmental stress levels, nutritional advances, and perhaps through hormonal tampering of the poultry and livestock which humans are consuming.

This last topic regarding the addition of anabolic hormones to the poultry and livestock will be discussed in detail in Part 6 of this book.

As previously mentioned, the pattern of growth hormone release is affected by many parameters. A comprehensive listing of substances or conditions which stimulate the release of growth hormone is contained in Table 9 below. A similar listing of the substances or conditions which inhibit the release of growth hormone within the body is contained in Table 10 on page 87. These extensive tables have been included for several reasons. First, they show that there has been substantial research in this area. Second, they point out the magnitude and variety of the known factors or molecules which will stimulate or inhibit growth hormone release within the body. Third, they serve as sources for further discussion and understanding. And, again, it is im-

Table 9: Growth Hormone Releasers

Extreme stress
Exercise
Sleep
Fasting
Hypoglycemia
Amino acid infusion (oral?)
Insulin administration
Growth hormone releasing hormone
Glucagon administration
Monoamines
    Dopamine receptor stimulators
        L-dopa
        bromoergocryptine
        Pribedil®
    Alpha-Adrenergic receptor stimulators
        amphetamines
        clonidine (Catapres®)
        epinephrine
        caffeine?
    Beta-Adrenergic receptor blockers
        propranolol (Inderal®)
    Serotonin precursors
        L-tryptophan
        5-hydroxytryptophan
    GABA and GABA receptor stimulators
    Cholinergic receptor stimulators
    Melatonin

(From Taylor, *Anabolic Steroids and the Athlete*, McFarland, 1982)

**Table 10: Substances or Conditions
That Inhibit Growth Hormone Secretion**

Somatostation
High serum hGH levels?
High serum somatomedin levels?
Hyperglycemia
Monoamines
 Dopamine agonists in certain diseases
  Bromoergocryptine
  Apomorphine
  Parlodel®?
 Alpha-Adrenergic blockers
  Phentolamine
  Phenoxybenzamine
  Minoxidil
 Antiserotonin agents
  Methysergide
  Periactin® (cyproheptadine)
  p-Chlorophenyalanine
 Beta-Adrenergic agonists
  Isoproteronol

(From Taylor, *Anabolic Steroids*, 1982)

portant to remember that much of this information listed in these two tables results from the extreme efforts of experimental medical physicians oriented toward a better understanding of the differential diagnosis and treatment of "slow-growing" children.

Before addressing specifically each of the substances which stimulates growth hormone release within the body, it is important to cover some of the basic physiological considerations of growth hormone release in an effort to further realize the importance of this phenomenon. Among the basic physiological conditions which stimulate growth hormone release are sleep, exercise, and extreme stress conditions.

Sleep

The amount of growth hormone released during the sleeping hours is usually greater than at any other time of the day. Usually, this growth hormone release is in a decrescendoing, peaking fashion throughout normal sleep. The initial peak is usually the largest release of growth hormone, and it occurs usually within the first 45 to 90 minutes of sleep. Typically, especially in younger people, there are several secondary peak releases of growth hormone which may occur during the later hours of sleep. These occur at approximately 90-minute intervals with a decreasing frequency and decreasing absolute peak release.

Within a given individual, almost every factor involved with the sleep-induced release of growth hormone may vary. These include:

• the absolute height of the initial hGH release;

• the presence or absence of the additional secondary peaks of hGH release;

• the frequency and absolute heights of these secondary hGH peaks.

Also of interest, it has been shown that either *aging* affects growth hormone release or that changes in growth hormone release account for major factors involved with the aging process of humans. For some unknown reason, the following changes occur with the sleep-induced release of growth hormone with advancing age:

(1) The initial absolute height of the growth hormone release during the first 45 to 90 minutes of sleep becomes significantly less and less until it eventually may discontinue altogether in elderly persons.

(2) The frequency and absolute heights of the secondary growth hormone peaks during the later stages of sleep become significantly less until they may discontinue in middle-aged and elderly persons.

Whether these reductions in the sleep-induced growth hormone releases cause aging, or whether aging in general results in this phenomenon is unknown at this time. But it is known that the anabolic mechanisms of growth hormone affect the repair mechanisms and immune systems of the body in a positive and protective fashion.

It may be that as persons age, the ability to sleep effectively reduces. To be sure, as people age and engage in life's stresses and injustices, the ability to "turn off" mentally and fall asleep effectively reduces, and thus more and more older people take sleeping medication on a clinical basis.

As an important aside, it has been shown convincingly that significant ethanol consumption in the evening prior to sleep tends to *blunt* the ensuing sleep-induced growth hormone release. In fact, in persons who chronically overconsume ethanol prior to sleep, the sleep-induced growth hormone release may completely disappear. In this extreme case, this phenomenon may ultimately play a significant role in the premature aging and early immune shutdown of alcoholics.

Therefore, it seems to be a logical conclusion that adequate and frequent growth hormone release during sleep is essential for continued youth and health.

Exercise

Exercise probably stimulates the release of growth hormone within the body by an indirect mechanism. With significant exercise, some of the body's monoamines and catecholamines, such as epinephrine and norepinephrine are released by the adrenal glands. Also, adrenocorticotropic hormone, ACTH, is released from the adrenal glands as well during exercise, and all of these molecules are known growth hormone releasers.

The specifics as to the quantity, quality and type of exercise which cause the most efficient, most consistent release of growth hormone are essentially unknown at this time. However, growth hormone release in response to exercise is an important part of the conditioning, repairing, and tissue-building responses. In fact, this exercise-induced release of growth hormone is probably at the crux of the physiological changes induced by proper athletic training.

There seems to be some evidence that this exercise-induced release of growth hormone is so variable that it may be difficult to study on a scientific basis. Some evidence suggests that interval training and altering the intensity of regular training may both be important factors in maintaining a sensitive exercise-induced growth hormone release. There also seems to be some evidence to suggest that the exercise-induced growth hormone release may be *the* important mechanism dealing with skeletal muscle hypertrophy and hyperplasia changes seen especially with weight training athletes on a longitudinal basis.

Extreme Stress

Probably by a similar mechanism as the exercise-induced release of growth hormone, extreme stress and perceived extreme stress causes a release in growth hormone. The catecholamines and ACTH are released during stressful or perceived stressful conditions, and again, these are known growth hormone releasers. My teachers always told me that stress would make me grow!

Exogenous Substances Which Cause hGH Release

Prior to discussing some of the substances which have been shown to cause a significant release of growth hormone within the body, it is important to cover further some basic concepts regarding growth hormone release. Many of these concepts make up the basis for which many people are currently using growth hormone releasers for body fat reduction and as an adjunct to their athletic regimen. These concepts are that:

• hGH has a very short half-life within the body (T½ of approximately 30 minutes);

• hGH release is multifactoral;

• hGH has only a short "refractory period" for which to inhibit further hGH release;

• hGH releasing stimuli combined together may result in further augmentation of hGH release.

Amino Acids

It is an unforgettable event to be serving as a medical officer for an international athletic event and be called to an athlete's room to start an intravenous line on this athlete for "dehydration" and subsequently watch the athlete push amino acid solutions into his body via the intravenous line. Not only did this occur in one particular athlete, but in several. Once the protective mechanism of the human skin is violated with a needle, the introduction of various substances into the body via this route can have astonishing effects.

Current medical research has shown that many of the known amino acids *infused* into an intravenous line into humans may result in a release of growth hormone from the pituitary gland similar to that release seen during sleep. Some of these amino acids include glycine, L-arginine, L-lycine, L-methionine, L-tryptophan, L-ornithine, and others. For instance, it has been shown that approximately *30 grams* of L-arginine for most men (15 grams for women) *infused* into an intravenous line causes a substantial release of growth hormone into the bloodstream. However, the exact amount of L-arginine taken by mouth which may cause a similar phenomenon is essentially unknown at this time. Extrapolation of this information is complicated by the following reasons:

(1) Whether or not a single amino acid taken orally will cause a significant release of growth hormone has not been studied to date. However, there is evidence to speculate that lower doses of a single amino acid may indeed cause a release of growth hormone, but probably well below the infused level.

(2) Whether or not smaller oral doses of two or more amino acids which are known to cause a growth hormone release will cause a significant release when taken together. Again, there is speculative evidence of the phenomenon only.

Two or more important aspects to consider regarding oral amino acid ingestion for augmenting growth hormone release are the quantity ingested and the time of ingestion. It is safe to say that the quantity of ingested amino acid probably releases growth hormone in a dose-related fashion. Current research also has shown that the timing of growth hormone stimulators is very important. Usually, when two or more of the known growth hormone stimulators (refer to Table 9) are combined together within an hour or so, the subsequent release of growth hormone will be greater than either of the single stimulators used alone. So, it may be that if amino acids in sufficient amounts are ingested slightly prior to a period of strenuous exercise, that the subsequent response of growth hormone release would be greater. This similar phenomenon has been well-documented with experiments on humans with L-dopa and Inderal®, with Catapres® and Inderal® and others. Another important time lending itself to possible growth hormone augmentation would be just prior to sleep. This combination of known growth hormone stimulators may indeed augment the normal response.

Improper timing of the combined or repeated stimuli for growth hormone release may result in a lack of the second stimulus to produce the effect. It seems as if there is a "refractory period" in which a second stimulus is applied during a period when growth hormone is *already elevated* then the second stimulus may not further release the hormone. This area of the control of human growth is in need of further study. And, it can be stated that this whole area of growth hormone releasers and stimuli is very complex and interesting.

Drugs

The most popular prescription drugs which athletes are currently using to enhance their growth hormone release are L-dopa, Catapres®, amphetamines, insulin and glucagon, the latter two by injection. As an example, a comparison of the serum growth hormone responses subsequent to hGH injection and to oral Catapres® are shown in Figure 3 on page 93. Oral Catapres® is an anti-hypertensive medication which is known to have a central alpha-2 agonist effect. It is currently the safest, most effective and most consistent releaser of growth hormone used in the clinical setting of provocative testing in children. Essentially, what is not known about the response of prolonged elevation of hGH is the subsequent responses of the liver to release the somatomedins, growth factors and multiplication factors. It is not known whether it is the peak hGH serum level or the total time of hGH serum elevation which is a more specific releaser of the somatomedins, growth factors and multiplication factors. This will be discussed later in this text.

Growth Hormone Releasing Hormone

As previously discussed, the hypothalamus secretes a polypeptide hormone, the growth hormone releasing hormone, which

**Figure 3: Comparison of the Serum Responses
to Oral Clonidine and Administered hGH**

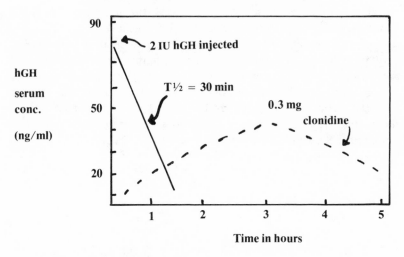

(From Taylor, *Anabolic Steroids*, 1982)

stimulates the pituitary gland to release human growth hormone into
the general blood stream. Recently, medical scientists have learned
how to identify, isolate, and produce this polypeptide hormone. Currently, there have actually been three amino acid sequences discovered
which function as growth hormone releasing hormones. One of these
has a known 29 amino acid sequence, another has a known 40 amino
acid sequence and a third has a known 44 amino acid sequence. It is
likely, that in the near future, large quantities of these analogs of
growth hormone releasing hormone, GHRH, with full biological
activity may be synthesized by recombinant-DNA genetic engineering
techniques similar to that used for human growth hormone. This
process should prove a more satisfactory and less expensive form of
therapy than exogenous human growth hormone administration for
some growth disorders. In addition, exogenous administration of
GHRH may allow a more natural preservation of the feedback mechanisms at the pituitary level, thereby resulting in a more physiological
approach for the induction of normal or supranormal growth. Furthermore, large doses of GHRH have been shown to be effective in
normal men if administered intranasally, such as a sniff of nasal spray,
thereby obviating the need for its injection.

The implications of this discovery are staggering and frightening if this type of hormone is misused. Essentially, GHRH *drives* the release of growth hormone, which has powerful effects on humans and animals as previously discussed. Obviously, this hormone, which will surely be synthesized in large quantities in the near future, will have an extremely high abuse potential, especially since it is active when sniffed. And, much like that of synthetic human growth hormone, it would have near untraceability with current drug testing procedures. Furthermore, once this hormone is mass-produced, it will be even more difficult to insure its proper use than even human growth hormone. Here again, the inertia of the science of good intentions could prove to be just the opposite if not properly controlled.

Summary and Discussion

The heading for this particular part contained a rather interesting concept, and after reading this part, the meaning of the heading should become more apparent. Essentially, scientific man, by learning to use his head, is controlling his head, at least the lower portions of it. The hypothalamus and pituitary glands are at the base of the brain, and we are indeed discovering how influential this base of the brain is.

If the drug controversy of the 1984 Olympic Games centered around the decade-old issue of anabolic steroids and the newly acclaimed human growth hormone, then the new wave of anabolic, ergogenic hormones may indeed be the growth hormone releasers, and more specifically, growth hormone releasing hormone. Certainly, if the reader still believes that we can dictate the morals of our athletes and future athletes by urine drug testing procedures, even as expensive as these procedures are, then it is possible that the major intent of this book has been missed. Indirectly, the reader should begin to realize that mankind is destined to tamper with his/her body via man-made hormones, and that control of such a practice must originate from assertive measures, not detective measures.

Traditionally, the International Olympic Committee (IOC) has listed a particular drug on its "banned" list only after a relatively accurate testing mechanism is established. Otherwise, what purpose would be served if a rule could not be enforced? The current estimate for the costs involved with urine testing the 1984 Olympic competitors has been reported to be over 2.5 million dollars. But, even this figure is attainable only by allowing for a substantial amount of volunteer help. In fact, if the (IOC) had to pay for the medical and professional volunteers involved with the testing of the athletes, and not just the ancillary testing costs, then drug testing would stop immediately. And, with the future wave of potential athletic enhancing hormones, the testing costs, if indeed testing is possible with antibody formation techniques or some other bizarre ultra-expensive method, the testing costs could easily be 10 million dollars or more. That is quite a large sum of money just to serve as a palliative measure!

In Part 5, another method of hormonal manipulation of athletes will be addressed. This next part will deal with another recent product of synthetic genius which must be "cultured," the somatomedins, or the workhorse molecules which are stimulated by elevated growth hormone levels. In other words, the pathway of hormonal manipulation will continue further into the thicket, possibly a crisis thicket of Andromeda magnitude. "The decision is in our hands," as Michael Crichton grimly states in *The Andromeda Strain*.

5

The Somato-
medin Breakthrough

Procrustes in modern dress, the scientist will prepare the bed on
which mankind must lie; and if mankind doesn't fit—well, that
will be just too bad for mankind. There will have to be some
stretching and amputations as have been going on ever since
applied science really got into its stride, only this time they will
be a good deal more drastic than in the past.... In *Brave New
World* this standardization of the human product has been pushed
to fantastic, though not impossible, extremes.

Aldous Huxley,
Brave New World (1946)

In Greek mythology Procrustes was a giant from Attica who
seized travelers and tied them to an iron bedstead, after which he
either cut off their legs or stretched his shorter victims until they fitted
it. In this manner Procrustes tortured his victims into conformity or
uniformity by drastic methods. One of the modern day methods to
force the human structure to uniformity may be through the widespread use of the somatomedins, and in this manner, what evolves
may be the Procrustean Society.

Introduction: The somatomedins may potentially unlock the doors to growth, longevity and a new world.

Recently, one of the most influential breakthroughs in medical science occurred in the area of growth and development of humans: the total synthesis of somatomedin-C, Sc. Previously medical scientists have had to be content with just measuring the somatomedin levels in the serum of humans who have normal growth, constitutionally rapid growth, and a variety of growth disorders. Historically, the tissue concentrations of the somatomedins have been so low that obtaining enough of them to study impeded the necessary research in this exciting area of medical endocrinology. And, as previously shown, many exciting areas of endocrinology seem to enter the athletic arena rather quickly.

In the first four parts of this book, several hormones and hormonal pathway considerations have been discussed from an athletic perspective. In the first two parts, the use of the analogs of the male sex hormone, testosterone, was considered. In the third and fourth parts, hormones, drugs and other stimuli which *drive* the growth of humans were discussed in some detail and then related to the athletic arena. And, in Part 5, another method of *driving* the human growth system via hormonal manipulation will be presented.

Previously, the importance of speculative science was discussed. And, the further one speculates from the current base of scientific knowledge, the more difficult it becomes to believe just what could occur via the passage of time.

At this point, the reader may be wondering why more physicians are not aware of the potential seriousness of some of this speculation from scientific facts. Indeed, is this book really just science fiction, or do these concepts based on scientific facts seem more strange than fiction itself? Well, in any area of human accomplishment, there will be parts of the pathway which are not well-trodden. Historically, many "pioneers" have been nothing more than ambitious managers of knowledge obtained from several disciplines of study. And, in some cases, after the "pioneer" has made the pathway accessible to others, then the people involved with the intertwined areas of study may envision what contributions came from their particular field of expertise. In this same manner, then, maybe this book will "pioneer" the experts in the fields of medical endocrinology to understanding the extent of potential abuse their genius represents.

The experimental research from the related fields of medical endocrinology is expanding at a rate which is unsurpassed by any area of medical research. For, when a new hormone is discovered, isolated, and synthesized, medical scientists are anxious to use the hormone in a wide variety of clinical settings. And, if these same scientists have several hormones to use concurrently, then the rate of knowledge expands nearly exponentially for the ensuing years. The more that is known about the complex hormonal network involved with human growth, the more complex the whole system seems to become, in some cases. However, as previously stated, this type of research is firmly entrenched in the evolution of mankind.

Somatomedins and "Selective Gigantism"

Overwhelming evidence that somatomedin-C is an obligate mediator of growth hormone action has been secured to a great degree. Somatomedin-C, also known as insulin-like growth factor-1, has a major role in controlling the cellular growth and maturation of humans. Somatomedin-C is controlled, at least in part, by the secretion of growth hormone, but it seems to be controlled physiologically by a number of other factors, including diet. And, to show the relative importance of this polypeptide molecule to human growth, it has recently been shown that the reason pygmies have such a short stature is that they have a relative lack of somatomedin-C. Furthermore, it may be that other ethnic groups with predominately short stature may have a relative lack of somatomedin-C or other growth factor.

Previously in Part 4 of this book, a schematic representation of the organs involved with the human growth hormone system was presented. And from this schematic, it can be shown that the somatomedin production occurs primarily in response to elevated growth hormone levels. These somatomedins are synthesized in the human body primarily by the liver, but also secondarily by the kidneys. In effect, the somatomedins are at the end of this anabolic system which can be stimulated in a multifactored manner.

In any current discussion regarding the piecemeal knowledge known about somatomedins and the role which somatomedins play in human growth, the depth of the discussion must be selected so that total confusion is not the result. However, when a topic is not considered in full detail, then some misconceptions may occur. Therefore, a relatively shallow approach to this topic will follow, but hopefully, this approach will mislead no one.

Once the somatomedins are released from the liver and possibly the kidneys, they exhibit a considerable anabolic effect on the tissues of the human body. At the present time, all of these anabolic effects are not known. However, a basic summary of the known effects of the somatomedins are:

In muscle: increased amino acid transport
increased protein synthesis
increased glucose transport intracellularly
increased formation of glycogen
potentiates mitosis of muscle cells

In cartilage: increased amino acid transport
increased synthesis of RNA and DNA
increased formation of proteoglycans
increased synthesis of collagen
potentiates cartilage cell mitosis

Therefore, from the above listing of some of the known effects of the somatomedins, it is safe to say that they have a tremendous anabolic effect on the human body.

As briefly mentioned above, the factors which alter the somatomedin levels in the serum are multifactored and not fully elucidated to date. There is some evidence that high levels of somatomedins in the serum have a negative feedback inhibition effect on the hypothalamus. In effect, then, one of the controlling factors of the somatomedin levels in the serum is the somatomedin level itself.

Before discussing some of the other controlling factors involved with the somatomedin serum level regulation, it is important to know how the somatomedins are carried by the bloodstream. They circulate in the plasma predominantly as a large molecular weight binding protein complex of 150,000 MW. Also, the plasma contains a smaller molecular weight binding protein of approximately 90,000 MW.

In general, the levels of the somatomedins and the large protein binding complex appear to be regulated primarily by growth hormone, but there are many exceptions to this generality. There seem to be several factors which may cause a temporary shift in the amount of "bound" somatomedin and "free" somatomedin, without actually exerting any control of the total serum concentration of somatomedins.

There is substantial evidence that some dietary components may play a regulatory role in the serum somatomedin-C concentrations in humans. Basically, conclusions are that both protein and energy intake (calories) serve as regulators of somatomedin-C concentrations in adult humans. And, there is some correlation between changes in the somatomedin-C concentrations and the total body nitrogen balance, which is considered a marker for anabolic ability. Of course, since it has been previously stated that proteins, and especially certain amino acids, cause a release in growth hormone, we would expect a subsequent rise in the somatomedin-C levels as well. That is how the pathway functions. However, all of the dietary components involved in the modulation of serum somatomedin concentrations in humans have not been defined.

Other factors which seem to alter the somatomedin levels in human serum are the sex hormones; however, all of the details of this controlling mechanism are unknown at this time. It has been shown that exogenous testosterone in boys can subsequently cause a rise in somatomedin levels. In some cases, exogenous progesterogenic steroids can give rise to increased levels of somatomedins.

During puberty, the greatest elevations of somatomedins are seen, with peak levels of over three times the level in normal adult serum. These highly elevated somatomedin-C levels are consistent with the rapid growth rates seen in puberty. These very high levels of somatomedins seem to be primarily controlled by the increases in pulsatile growth hormone surges from the pituitary gland.

To further the complexity of the entire scope of the regulatory control of the somatomedin levels, there is some evidence that there are actually some somatomedin inhibitors in the serum. There is also a theory to suggest that it is the balance between the somatomedins and the somatomedin inhibitors which ultimately controls the anabolic responses. However, this concept is in need of further study.

Therefore, from the aforementioned discussion, it is safe to say that medical science is busy piecing the somatomedin control puzzle together, and that it is at least as complex as the control mechanisms of human growth hormone. However, with the newly synthesized somatomedin-C, much of this complex control arrangement should be worked out in detail.

So, how does all of this information shed light on the potential athletic use or misuse of the future mass-produced somatomedin-C? Well, one of the most interesting findings in children who are "labeled" as *constitutionally tall*, is that their somatomedin-C levels are consistently higher than that of children who are predicted to reach normal ranges of adult height. Constitutionally-tall children and adolescents will ultimately be taller than the normal range of adult height. And, in these same children and adolescents, the increased somatomedin-C levels seem to stem from increased growth hormone release.

Therefore, it appears that by *driving* the human growth pathway in some manner height increases will result; and in fact, that is how giants are made biologically. Speculative ways to *drive* this human growth pathway in a growing child destined to excel in athletics could probably be accomplished in the following manners:

(1) by chronic injections or chronic intranasal administration of growth hormone releasing hormone or its analogs;

(2) by chronic injections of synthetic human growth hormone;

(3) by chronic injections of synthetic somatomedin-C;

(4) by chronic stimulation of the hypothalamus via drugs, amino acids or other stimuli to enhance the release of growth hormone releasing hormone;

(5) some combination of methods (1) through (4) above.

Another interesting phenomenon deals with the "wearing-out" effect of the human pituitary gland and physiological aging. Previously, in Part 4, the topic of growth hormone release was considered. And, it was stated that as humans age, the rejuvenating pulses of growth hormone release diminish in number and peak height. This means, that as we age, we have much less growth hormone release to carry out the required anabolic functions. Recently, it has been shown that the primary reason for this is that the pituitary gland tends to release less and less growth hormone in the face of a strong stimulus to release more. In effect, the somatotrophic cells of the anterior portion of the pituitary gland must wear out in some age-related fashion. So, by knowing this finding, if one were to maintain a "youthful" growth hormone releasing pattern, could we delay aging? To date, this is the strongest concept for anti-aging ever considered. And, it may be possible to maintain this "youthful" anabolic potential of the human growth system by several mechanisms:

(1) by enhanced stimuli to the somatotrophic cells of the anterior pituitary gland to produce growth hormone physiologically. This could be accomplished by using growth hormone releasing hormone or by using selected drugs or conditions to augment the growth hormone releasing hormone levels;

(2) by directly injecting synthetic growth hormone on a chronic basis;

(3) by injecting somatomedin-C on a chronic basis;

(4) or by some combination of the methods listed above.

Summary and Discussion

This part of the book, although shorter in length than the preceding parts, gives us some clues to where mankind under the influence of scientific momentum may be led. It also gives the reader some insight in dealing with the molecular make-up of the human body. As we find more molecules, we ultimately find more molecules! It also replants the idea that hormonal manipulation of our bodies, whether it be under the auspices of enhanced athletic potential or not, is coming.

Traditionally, we have looked to history for clues to whether or not divine intervention, or in my personal case, God, actually created mankind. By delving into this topic, it is difficult to believe that man could have evolved in such a complex molecular biological manner, without beginning there for the most part. It is very difficult to imagine that with all of the proposed millions of years dealing with the evolutionary history of mankind, we would have not begun with most of the complex physiological pathways which we have now. In effect, the system we have now for securing normal growth has extreme measures for checks and balances, that is, until we begin the continuing saga of hormonal manipulation!

Learning about our biological being and formulating the molecules which may treat or prevent disease are definite benefits of profound study. We must never forget that man is curious about himself, and, in many areas, the more man learns, the more man can learn. But learning must be in a controlled environment, especially when the topic to be learned affects the whole of society. And, with a substantial percentage of our society involved with self-experimentation with anabolic steroids and human growth hormone via the well-established black market sources, it does not require much speculation to envision a major problem with synthetic somatomedin-C.

Since somatomedin-C has only recently been synthesized, any discussion of the potential adverse conditions which may afflict the athletic user of the hormone would necessarily be based on theory and speculation at this point. An obviously potential adverse effect would be *athletic acromegaly* with many of the same potential adverse effects of overproduction of or exogenously administered human growth hormone. However, there may be several unforeseen adverse conditions associated with chronic somatomedin-C use such as antibody formation against itself or even the possibility of cancer in the tissues in which it stimulates growth.

The development of commercial products through the use of advanced biological science, especially recombinant-DNA and advanced mutational techniques, is the primary interest of a Swiss company, Biogen. Through a joint venture with KabiVitrum AB, also of Switzerland, Biogen expects to market synthetic human somatomedin-C (recombinantly produced) for treating growth disorders, skeletal muscle atrophy, bone fractures and for burn and wound healing by 1988. Biogen has pilot plant facilities in Cambridge, Massachusetts which include fermenters large enough to produce sufficient product for clinical trials and marketing purposes.

To think that this powerful genetically-engineered human anabolic molecule would not lend itself to athletic misuse and abuse is certainly tunnel vision. And, due to the previous discussion presented in this part, as well as the remainder of the text, I must continue to recommend that *all* of the anabolic hormones synthesized by recombinant-DNA genetic-engineering techniques be classified as highly controlled drugs by the FDA prior to their release on mankind. Otherwise, we are again reduced to the mythological methods of Procrustes, where the pulling and stretching of the human body by these molecules will be drastic torture indeed!

6

Nonathletic Hormonal Manipulation: Treating Pseudo-Disease Conditions

Introduction

In the previous five parts of the book, the current and future wave of anabolic hormones available for enhancing athletic skills has been examined. And, if locker room semantics refers to anabolic steroids as the "roids," then the future manipulation of athletes with a variety of anabolic hormones may eventually be referred to as the "mones."

Most of us wish that the athlete with the most natural ability who trains with the greatest intensity and who is the smartest will, in most circumstances, dominate athletic excellence. Unfortunately, anabolic hormones may be necessary to restore an equal competition under the current international conditions. Simply put, I am afraid that athletes can never go back to the pre-anabolic hormone era, and in a sense, mankind has lost some of its most profound innocence. Will this ultimately blunt our quest to place selected athletes in the roles of legends and invulnerable heroes? That is, now that we all know that anabolic hormones are the breakfast of champions!

For persepctive's sake, it may be beneficial to glance back at mythology. A hero of the famed *Iliad* was Achilles, who was the mythological answer to the modern bodybuilding superathlete, except for his "Achilles heel." As the legend goes, he was a "bowed-up" man who was held by the heel and dipped into the river Styx, which gave him an unusually thick skin except for the unsubmerged heel, which was later pierced by an arrow shot by Paris. Achilles died at the age of twenty-two, and his choice in life was to "roar like a lion" for his short life, instead of a lifelong sheep-like grazing existence which conduces greater longevity. But Achilles had the choice to make, and he selected to "roar like a lion." As a corollary, most of the competitive athletes whom I have had the opportunity to converse with would also choose to "roar like a lion" even at the risk of a shortened life span. Even "life span" is a risky term, for one's span cannot be determined until death, and then it is too late to weigh the risks and benefits of anything. And historically, cultures have always been able to find legendary heroes who by one means or another have made themselves invulnerable.

Maybe our idealistic American dream of fair play cannot apply to competitive athletics on an international basis. In world class competitive athletics, the situation may be far removed from fair play. And, in many cases, to beat them, you must join them. Just maybe, we have instilled in our people the concept that life's pleasures are derived from achieving goals—for in this sense most people will do almost anything to achieve success. So, from this point of view, the reward-oriented athlete quickly realizes that to achieve the goal in many areas of competitive sports, anabolic hormones may be a necessity. And in this case, the ends may indeed justify the means. But, really only the athlete can make this decision for his/her life.

The athletic arena is not the only area inflicted with hormonal manipulation with controversial intentions. In this part of the book, other methods of altering people and their expressive natures by hormonal manipulation will be briefly discussed. Hopefully, by including this part, the reader can further place the hormonal manipulation of athletes into the proper perspective. A careful examination of the material presented in this part may further erode the reader's faith in ethical and moral stances previously constructed.

Altering Human Expression by Administered Hormones

In a simple-to-perform experiment which was shown to me, sprinkling a crushed-up oral anabolic steroid tablet into an aquarium full of fish causes some interesting changes in the appearances and behaviors of the fish. The male fish's colors heighten and so does its aggressive behavior. The male *and* female fish may ultimately become violent and kill each other. Along these same lines, I once knew a young man who became enthralled in tropical fish fights augmented by the alterations in mood afforded by anabolic steroid administration to the aquarium water in which the fish lived.

The most fabulous ocean shell collection I ever saw belonged to an elderly, scientifically-oriented male nurse. He lives on an area of the gulf coast of Florida known as the "miracle strip." After the violent ocean storms and hurricanes which frequent this area, he would scan the beach and shallow waters along the beach in search of various types of still-living shellfish. He would gather them and quickly place them into his large saltwater aquarium. He would then administer anabolic steriods to this aquarium, and the shellfish and shell dwellers would respond to this milieu of anabolic steroid-enhanced saltwater by greater coloring in the shells.

An intense electrician whom I had the opportunity to work with during a summer vacation between my medical school years used to fight and breed "pit" bulldogs. He won by manipulating these vicious dogs with anabolic steroids to afford them greater muscle mass and strength, as well as the aggressive, violent nature needed to destroy the other dog.

During my medical internship, I met a surgeon who used anabolic steroids to manipulate his farm animals and race horses. He seemed to think that this phenomenon was common among knowledgeable farmers and horse breeders.

Of course, these types of lower animal manipulation by hormones cannot be directly extrapolated to humans—or can they? Physicians and medical scientists seem to be exploring the outer limits of medical ethics with a variety of highly questionable indications for the manipulation of people via hormonal tampering. Some of these situations will be listed and discussed below.

Hormonal "Stunting" of Growth for Constitutionally Tall Girls

During the past few years, physicians have "coined" a type of growth disorder of girls who will actually grow to heights of over six feet. However, whether being considered too tall as a treatable disorder or not is highly controversial, especially without some substantial reason. Excessive height may present a psychological dilemma for a young girl, and in many cases, tall girls have some degree of spinal curvature (scoliosis) which may be worsened by excessive height. Proposed therapies for this condition include repeated use of high-dose estrogenic steroids or drugs such as bromocriptine which are blockers of growth hormone release. These therapies, if begun during the rapid growth phases of puberty, can ultimately shorten the girl's height several inches according to current theories. However, while medical scientists are attempting to unravel all of the potential physical adverse conditions associated with this type of hormonal manipulation, and there are some, the ethical and philosophical issues seem to have been ignored.

Furthermore, as has been previously stated in this book, any significant hormonal manipulation usually is accompanied by alteration of the mental make-up in an unpredictable fashion. Who should receive this type of hormonal manipulation while the girl is yet a minor? Who will determine this? Who has the right to determine this? What are we altering, heights or heads? How is this concept any different than hormonally manipulating athletically-inclined children? Could physicians utilize these techniques to create the perfect jockey for winning large sums of money? Wouldn't this be giving hormones to healthy persons? Could physicians use this concept to make the perfect short gymnastic performer? Why isn't everyone outraged by this type of hormonal manipulation?

Another relatively common method of hormonally manipulating the growth patterns of young children desirous of future athletic endeavors is via the use of the progesterogenic steroid hormone, medroxyprogesterone. In athletic vernacular, this type of hormone is referred to as a "brake drug," for if administered to young girls who require a smallish stature for competitive gymnastics, the childhood years tend to be prolonged and the effects of puberty are blocked. This type of "childhood suspension" is felt to be common in the East Bloc countries, and some knowledgeable sporting figures feel that this may become a problem in the United States. How would parents in this country view this bizarre method of "childhood suspension" in their daughters?

It may be that international athletic competition would force some people to make some poor judgments as parents, since the rewards are great, aren't they?

Hormonal Inhibition of Pregnancy

H.G. Wells, in *Mind at the End of Its Tether* (1946), has noted that "Nature in her insensate play with the possibilities of life has produced some abrupt novelties in the record by accelerating the fertilization and ripening of the ovum relatively to the other phases of the life cycle."

It should seem obvious that indefinitely preventing normal functions which Nature has allowed for is basically incorrect. Furthermore, stopping Nature is difficult and usually results in some obvious, and sometimes unforeseen, adverse effects.

Millions of women take the birth control pill in this country. And, without dwelling on this topic, it is indeed hormonal manipulation of otherwise healthy young women. It is safe to say that women who take prescribed hormones to prevent pregnancy are flirting with some great risks, such as strokes, liver cancer, blood clots, body weight and body fat gains, breast cancer, cervical cancer and so on. This method of hormonal manipulation of healthy persons has significantly influenced the moral milieu of our society. So, in effect, it is socially acceptable to inhibit pregnancy, even with known adverse effects, by allowing women the right to take excessive quantities of female hormones. How is this different than men taking male hormones?

Is society saying that preventing pregnancy is acceptable, but achieving athletic excellence is not, even if both are products of hormonal manipulation? Since I personally feel that prescribing birth control pills is overtly dangerous, and owing to the fact that I have personally had to care for two teen-age girls who suffered strokes and two young women dying of liver cancer who took the birth control pill, I have refrained from ever prescribing them.

In other words, a woman asks to be hormonally manipulated to prevent pregnancy, and most physicians will grant this request. But, if an athlete asks for a similar type of hormonal manipulation to enhance athletic performance, the same physician will usually deny this request and offer an assortment of invalid excuses. Are we entering the age of the continuing saga of *selective* hormonal manipulation? I might add that I have discussed this topic with some athletes who were keenly aware of the risks and benefits of what they were asking for, but I have never discussed the risks and benefits of the birth control pill with a woman who was as well informed about what she was requesting. Again, why is there such a stigma associated with the use of anabolic hormones for enhancing athletic performance of persons who wish to engage in this type of therapy? Which is more important, athletic achievement or pregnancy? Does the eye of the beholder mean anything? Does it seem intrinsically safer to totally inhibit a normal body function (pregnancy) or to simply enhance some normal body functions (muscle development)? What if physicians halted the trend to freely prescribe estrogenic/progesterogenic steroids for birth control? Don't you feel that if this occurred a "black market" for the birth control pill would then arise? Furthermore, and perhaps more directly pertinent, some research groups are beginning to discover that even some types of birth control medications actually enhance athletic performance in women athletes. However, these types of birth control hormones are "legal" for all levels of athletic competition.

Chemical Castration of Rapists

The use of Depo-Provera®, which is an injectable progesterogenic steroid hormone, has been investigated for use in convicted rapists to "cure" them from their uncontrollable habits of raping, and usually mentally destroying, a woman. Apparently, the proposed mechanism is to block the effects of the male hormone testosterone which controls the sexual desires of both men and women to a great degree. Hopefully, this concept, which will be in the control of physicians if accepted, is as sound as the proponents suggest, for if it is not, then we will have to suffer the horrible events which may follow clinical failure. In other words, this would allow the rapist to rape another woman and potentially destroy the hopes and dreams of a woman and her family.

Again, this is an excellent example of using the body's own hormonal system to alter subsequent human expressions and actions. In effect, this concept of chemical castration for convicted rapists relies on blocking the effects of one hormone with another hormone exogenously given. And, since this essentially is a balancing between the two hormones to inhibit sexual desire, what is to keep the freed convicted rapist from obtaining black market anabolic steroids to administer to himself without the knowledge of the physician in charge of providing the rapist with his monthly Depo-Provera® injections? Nothing! Aren't some rapists athletes and bodybuilders anyway? Do they rape while under the influence of the anabolic steroids? These are important issues, for certain.

Hormonally "Padding" the Farmer's Wallet

Accusations involving the use by farmers and feed producers of hormones to increase the body weight and growth rate of farm animals are certainly not new ones. Apparently, there is enough residual hormone in the meat and other products subsequently ingested by humans to alter their own hormonal balances. For instance, an epidemic of premature thelearche, with over 2000 young girls from Puerto Rico and the Caribbean islands, continues to be of great concern. Premature thelearche is essentially premature breast development and enlargement in girls prior to the age of 8 years or so. Researchers concluded that estrogenic steroid contamination of the animal feed was associated with the cause of this phenomenon. Furthermore, a large percentage of these young girls showed signs of precocious puberty as young as 2 years of age. These signs included growth of pubic hair, onset of menstruation and advanced bone development, which may ultimately shorten their stature significantly. One of the researchers was reported to have had her car "fire-bombed" shortly after disclosing this information.

In another incident, Italian physicians have reported that a condition in epidemic numbers of gynecomastia has been associated with estrogenic steroid hormone contamination or addition to the feed supply of the farm animals. Gynecomastia is abnormal breast development in males, and in this case, young boys attending an Italian school near Milan.

According to current United States standards, there are *limits* to the quantities of anabolic hormones which may be added to the feed for animals intended for subsequent human consumption. What this really indicates is that the government feels safe to allow some hormonal manipulation of these harvested animals, but not too much. How much is too much? Well, again this depends on various types of testing procedures performed on the meat end-product and the intent, accuracy, and consistency of the testing. It also seems to rely on exactly who is doing the testing; and for the Puerto Rico epidemic cited above, there are claimed extreme differences in the amount of end-product hormone concentrations. Essentially, government testing passes, but private testing shows very high concentrations of anabolic hormones in the meat. And, any food product that can cause a two year-old toddler to develop breasts, pubic hair and menstrual cycles is a real threat to the present health of the child. Furthermore, such premature development is most likely to have some effects on the ultimate growth and development of the child as she reaches later stages in life. Is a similar type of low-grade hormonal manipulation of livestock practiced in the United States? How would we know? Are the Third World countries just experiments? We know that some of the major pharmaceutical companies have supplied large amounts of anabolic steroids as "appetite stimulators" to some Third World countries. Why not just "doctor" the food products as well? Isn't this similar to what Hitler had in mind?

There is definitely an interest in developing giant farm animals. Experiments targeted at increasing the growth rate and subsequent adult size of farm animals has come under attack by an opponent of genetic engineering and an animal protectionist. Jeremy Rifkin of the Foundation of Economic Trends and Michael W. Fox of the Humane Society of the United States have filed a suit in a United States District Court to halt experiments involving the transfer of the human growth hormone gene into farm animals. There is good supportive evidence that human growth hormone produced by such a gene in farm animals will create gigantic animal specimens. In the scientific literature recently, a study indicated that agricultural application of the human growth hormone gene into mice caused the mice to produce human growth hormone and grow to be twice the size of normal mice. Further trials using the human growth hormone gene, similar to that used both in these mice and in the bacterial vats which produce synthetic human growth hormone, are eventually planned to be carried out using livestock.

In recent years, many hundreds of embryos of pigs and sheep have been injected with the human growth hormone gene, and about 50 animals are being tested to determine whether the gene is present in these growing animals, and whether the gene is functioning within the animals, forcing them to make human growth hormone. It has been previously pointed out that human growth hormone tends to be active in lower animals.

The plaintiffs are claiming that transferring genetic material between animal species is a violation of the moral and ethical potential of civilization. Furthermore, they contend it poses a grave potential threat to the biological integrity of each species, and represents a new and insidious form of cruelty toward animals. But, the major concept in question is whether the transferring of a synthetic copy of the human DNA (growth hormone gene) is the same thing as taking the genetic material from a human and placing it into an animal. The former approach has been apparently approved by the appropriate committee involved, the recombinant DNA advisory committee of the National Institutes of Health.

The entire scope of genetically-engineered growth in humans to potentially cause "selective gigantism" and in farm animals to cause gigantic livestock specimens seems overwhelming. However, it has been a long, stepwise series of scientific experiments. When medical science placed the human growth hormone gene into bacterial cultures to synthesize human growth hormone, no one was worried about the bacteria's status or health. But, when the similar techniques are used to inject farm animal embryos, we hear opposition from the Humane Society. My concerns are for the human being, and if these series of scientific experiments continue, will the human embryo be next? And all of this under the auspices of scientific advancement? Is scientific advancement, more specifically recombinant-DNA genetic engineering, outstripping our abilities to legislate effectively? What attorney, or better yet, what man of any profession can legislate these types of advancements appropriately enough to insure that the products will be of benefit to mankind, instead of destroying the species integrity and everything in between. The creatures posed in the *Return of the Jedi* may be just waiting in the wings!

Summary and Discussion

In this part of the book other areas in which the infiltration of hormones into nonathletic circumstances has been presented. Only a few selected areas have been shown in this book, for the major thrust of this material has been directed toward the athletic use of anabolic hormones and the surrounding circumstances of this phenomenon. However, by considering some corollary concepts, the reader may gain a more complete understanding of the complexity and powers of hormonal manipulation. Also, the reader should begin to realize that whether the topic is athletic training, or preparing for an athletic role in a motion picture, or legislating the morality of convicted rapists, or altering the growth rate of the entire country, hormonal manipulation may be a major parameter in the discussion.

Hormonal manipulation will continue to be inflicted on mankind, and in some ways mankind has been lucky already, or has it? With such widespread use of the birth control pill, just what if there were some serious adverse effects which were not yet foreseen? Or what if the adverse conditions were tainted in such a manner that some government officials were deciding the "risks versus benefits" for you? In a sense, the widespread use of the birth control pill has been the most marked method of legislating morals and customs ever introduced. Will "selective gigantism" follow the same pathway in the evolution of mankind? Who *will* decide?

> Projects of the future will be vast government-sponsored inquiries into what the politicians and the participating scientists will call "the problem of happiness" — in other words, the problem of making people love their servitude.... First, a greatly improved technique of suggestion — through infant conditioning and, later, with the aid of drugs....
>
> Aldous Huxley, *Brave New World* (1946)

> This country supports the largest scientific establishment in the history of mankind. New discoveries are constantly being made, and many of these discoveries have important political or social overtones. In the near future, we can expect more crises on the pattern of Andromeda. Thus I believe it is useful for the public to be made aware of the way in which scientific crises arise, and are dealt with.
>
> Michael Crichton, *The Andromeda Strain* (1969)

Some of the scientific and medical implications of that prophecy are of major concern to Dr. Paul Berg, 1980 Nobel laureate and the so-called father of recombinant-DNA genetic engineering. In a late fall 1984 symposium, he made several concerning statements which could have easily flowed from the speculative-science pen of Michael Crichton such as: "I can see the potential for this information to intrude on personal freedoms.... Conceivably, the government could use this information to mandate how and where we live.... These possibilities raise a very important question: Do we really want all this information? ... scientists have created a monster [to] manipulate genes in a way which dehumanizes us.... [however, I] violently oppose efforts to restrict research" (*Medical World News*, November 12, 1984).

We need to develop a consensus about how far we wish genetic engineers to invade our personal lives, our bodies, and our humanity. What we need is rational decisions regarding the present *and* future of genetic engineering, and to inform the public in such a manner that they can enjoy the benefits of well-informed prophecy for the human race. This book aims at doing just that, for the first real horror which has sprung from this type of "gene crossing" is the athletic abuse potential of human growth hormone, and the near-future abuse potential of the other anabolic hormones synthesized by these techniques of combining human genetic material with other species.

And, until this consensus is reached after hearing from interdisciplinary experts, it obviously makes sense to *place anabolic hormones under strict control by the FDA.*

7

Conclusions: Stretching the Hippocratic Oath or Legislated Morality?

I will prescribe regimen for the good of my patients according to my ability and my judgment and never do harm to anyone. To please no one will I prescribe a deadly drug.

From the *Hippocratic Oath*

A series of events has forced upon the intelligent observer the realization that the human story has already come to an end and that *Homo sapiens*, as he has been pleased to call himself, is in his present form played out. The stars in their courses have turned against him and he has to give place to some other animal better adapted to face the fate that closes in more and more swiftly upon mankind.

That new animal may be an entirely alien strain, or it may arise as a new modification of the *hominidae*, and even as a direct continuation of the human phylum, but it will certainly not be human.... To many of us this crude alternative is intensely unpalatable. The forces that evolved us in the long succession of living beings endowed us with a tenacity of self-assertion that rebels against the bare idea of giving place to rats or unclean intrusive monsters equipped with streptococci for our undoing. We want to be in at the death of Man and to have a voice in his final replacement, even if, that successor's first act be parricide.

H.G. Wells, *The Mind at the End of Its Tether* (1946)

Introduction

"Parricide" is a little-used term for a person who murders either or both of his parents or someone else who stands to him in a somewhat similar relationship, and the best known of all parricides was Oedipus. According to legend, Oedipus was driven by the insatiable desire "to know," and this overwhelming desire enthralled him in a situation where he unknowingly killed his father and married his mother. And as a combined corollary, are we entering an era of polypeptide-induced parricide for mankind? Will the quest "to know" turn the modern medical scientist into an Oedipus-like genetic engineering genocidist or a species-combining genius? Somehow, this concept resembles the creation of Dr. Frankenstein all over again!

In the previous parts of this book, an extreme effort has been put forth to firmly entrench in the mind of the reader that the merging of science and athletics is not always a smooth or beneficial one. In fact, what may ultimately stem from the clashes of medical science and athletics may not be beneficial for humanity. However, it seems imperative at this time to apply some caution regarding the direction in which we may be headed, for taking a phenomenon such as this marriage on faith alone may prove to be destructive in nature.

One of the most difficult lines for me to draw is the "line" between faith and laziness. Ultimately, many times even the most assertive persons must rely on the powers of faith after they have done all that could be done. However, the fact that humans tend toward the lazy approach to issues sometimes leads us to leave to faith what otherwise could have been solved by profound study. And, many times, what we leave to faith fails for this exact reason. Therefore, the directions which modern medical science will afford us should not be taken on faith, but with profound study.

In this final part, the hypothetical views of many of the parties involved with the complex issues previously discussed will be addressed. However, after considering all of the various viewpoints, the question of where to place the liability of overt and covert mistakes will not be obvious to anyone. After all, this book has been predicated on the fact that this issue will be a continuum with a firm evolutionary basis.

As previously ascertained, the number of persons caught in this web of conflicting interests is significant. These persons include the athlete, parents of the athlete, coaches, black market distributors, private enterprise marketeers, the medical scientist, the physician and the medical lawmakers. Some of the more pertinent aspects of the stands which each of these people harbor will be reviewed next.

The Athlete

The athlete, owing to a variety of reasons, generally dissembles about his/her use of anabolic hormones. The athlete usually feels that if he/she confesses to this drug use, then any success which the athlete has will be directly attributed to the drugs and not to other aspects of training. The athlete is frustrated because sports medicine does not seem to have any of the answers on this complex issue. Most athletes feel that, if the adverse conditions which may occur are real ones, then they will occur in someone else. And, the athlete denies any of the psychological changes which the anabolic steroids cause. Furthermore, the athlete may have to engage in illegal distribution of the anabolic hormones to fellow athletes to gain enough remuneration to pay for his/her own use.

Some athletes prefer to take the anabolic hormones as a matter of course, while other athletes take them just to compete. Many athletes feel that taking these drugs away from them infringes on their rights. Most athletes who are knowledgeable in the area of anabolic hormones realize that these drugs will continue to play a role in athletics.

The Parent

The parent of the athlete who is using or contemplating the use of anabolic steroids for their believed enhancing abilities to the athletic body, is usually misinformed and unaware of the condition. Most parents display extreme mixed feelings toward this issue, for not only do they want their son or daughter to excel in athletics, but also they want them healthy as well. Some parents favor the use of anabolic hormones for their children. Many parents become angry when they are approached about the issue. Misinformed as they are, parents still represent a major role in directing the education of minor children. Becoming angry and denying this issue will not help matters.

The Coach

Coaches are generally held in very high esteem by the young athlete, and the athlete tends to place considerable value on what the coach says. The conflicts for the coach stem from trying to maintain a winning team or winning athletic program without misleading the athletes. Many times the pressures placed on the coach to win cloud his/her otherwise proper judgment. However, once anabolic steroids are introduced into a particular athletic program, the use of them increases dramatically. The coach is usually aware of the anabolic steroid use among the athletes, but it is not unusual for the coach to deny this. It is difficult for him to be a policeman, detective, and coach at the same time, and still win.

The Black Market Distributor

The black market distributor of anabolic steroids to athletic-oriented persons usually has secure intrinsic rationalization mechanisms to justify his activity and to protect his inner feelings. He will tell you that alcohol is unhealthy and that anabolic hormones are healthy. He will insist that it is more dangerous to participate in contact sports than to use anabolic steroids. He will quickly inform you about the perils of tobacco and obesity, and he will place these evils into perspective and compare them to anabolic steroid use. He will deny that the particular drugs he sells ever filter down to children. What is the most important aspect of the drug issue in sports to him is the size of his wallet. Like any other illegal drug dealer, he is cautious and sly. He may brag about how many drug inspectors he has bribed. He usually dislikes parents, for they are not direct customers, but he will take great pleasure in securing a piece of their paycheck so that their offspring can manipulate their bodies with the drugs. He can destroy years of parenting in a single sitting.

The Private Enterprise Marketeers

In many ways, for the private enterprise marketeers, it is money over morals and ethics in a total way. Unlike the black market distributor, the private enterprise marketeer does not have substantial internal rationalization methods in this issue. He cannot hear that the genius of science, which he is marketing to other uninformed, sometimes wealthy persons, may have potential harmful effects on people. He just does not want to know this, for it makes his financial scheme appear less attractive. He is quick to promote the concepts of free enterprise, for they help him make money. His equation does not allow for moral and ethical parameters, for he is a salesman. He hears and believes only what is needed to sell. If you "lay" morals and ethics on him, he will just wait a few days and call you again.

One of the current investment companies which is backing the surge of recombinant-DNA genetically engineered hormones and other similar products is Dean, Whitter & Reynolds Company. And, for individuals who have grossed over $200,000 for the past two consecutive years, they offer a substantial tax shelter investment for qualified persons who will invest $50,000 or more. So from this information, it becomes rather easy to expect that many prospective wealthy investors may not be attuned to the potential perils in which they are investing. Folks, this type of investing is considerably more encompassing than buying a house or some land somewhere. And, I hope that the investors realize that, in effect, if things go wrong, they may be investing in a potentially overwhelming destructive force directed at the genesis of mankind as a species.

The Medical Scientist

The medical scientist must "publish or perish." In many areas of investigational research, the scientist is unaware of all of the potential ramifications of his discoveries. He wishes to discover things that are beneficial for mankind, but once his inventions leave his control, they may be used in a manner differing from the wishes of the medical scientist. The medical scientist is usually approachable on the topics of ethics and morals. His philosophy is always worth considering, however, as many medical scientists have trouble relating to the problems of people. They are always idealistic and interesting people. Many medical scientists devote their entire lives to a single area of deep research.

The Practicing Physician

As a young physician enters his practice, he is much like an engineer, for it is often claimed that *engineering is where science gets down to work!* However, the practice of medicine is far from a science. And, in many cases, the practicing physician's knowledge in a specialized area of medicine is so limited that he must remember to "do no harm" and admit that he does not know.

The most appropriate way in which to describe the inner feelings of a concerned physician is contained in a statement which is attributed to Gandhi: "Imperfect ourselves, we must be tender toward others."

The physician usually is misinformed about athletic use of anabolic steroids. He usually avoids the issue when an athlete confronts him about his/her desire to use anabolic hormones. The physician oftimes feels "used." He is concerned about the overall health of the athlete, not just his/her athletic skills. Many times, after trying to educate the athlete to the risks and the benefits of anabolic hormones, and the athlete chooses to use the anabolics, the physician is frustrated and feels as though he has failed the athlete by not convincing him/her to avoid the drugs. Most physicians wish that anabolic hormones had no role in athletics. The physician usually has difficulty with understanding the athletic version of "winning at all costs." He may become angry when approached about the issue. The physician usually harbors thoughts that anabolic hormone use by athletes will be harmful to some athletes, and indeed, this may be true. For the physician, who has of late been taught to provide the risks and benefits of medical procedures and drugs, the difficulties in informing athletes concerning these risks or benefits stem from a specific lack of knowledge about these areas. Furthermore, with the anabolic hormone issue in athletics the physician is really not in control of the drug use. It is and has been out of his hands and in the hands of an assortment of nonprofessionals.

In summary, any option open to the physician regarding the anabolic steroid and anabolic hormone issue in athletics can be criticized. Any option which he chooses may result in breaking the Hippocratic Oath, which in effect instructs the physician to "first, do no harm!"

Within the next decade, we indeed will face the pathway leading to the continuing saga of hormonal manipulation. There is simply no doubt about it. Will this responsibility fall within the realm of the physician? I thought that the general public was tired of physicians "playing God." And, I doubt if physicians will accept the responsibilities associated with the surge of recombinant-DNA genetically engineered hormones. Furthermore, I doubt if physicians, or anyone else, can appropriately handle these responsibilities and liabilities, especially when they have "fallen from grace." I just do not see how the public can indiscriminately sue physicians who they will again ask to become "gods" in the near future.

The Drug Testing Official

Many sporting officials involved with anabolic hormone use by athletes believe that the problem can be solved with drug testing measures alone; it cannot. For some of these sporting officials, dependence on this approach alone tends to be a self-serving, "hand-washing" technique to avoid the issue. They are quick to report any type of literature on the newer hormones, which they cannot test for, that tends to indicate they may not enhance athletic performance. These officials tend to become preoccupied with testing adult athletes at the peak of their competitive years, and tend to discount the idea that the elite athlete often has had the advantages of the drugs for many years and can still test "clean." However, in my opinion, the proper use of drug testing measures is essential if sports really wants to rid itself of widespread use of performance-enhancing drugs.

Modern approaches to drug testing of selected athletes have brought negative results. In my opinion, they are:

• The general public and average sports fans have been misled as to who is actually using drugs, primarily testosterone and human growth hormone of late. They tend to believe that "clean" urine is synonymous with "drug free"; of course, it is not.

• The athletic careers and nationalistic pride of dozens of athletes have been destroyed; they have been "sacrificial lambs."

• The testing procedure has proven itself so far to be expensive and ineffective as a means of discouraging widespread use of anabolic hormones among athletes.

• The amount of paranoia among athletes and "athletic representatives" has dramatically increased, especially at international meets where a language barrier is present. Many athletes are misinformed at international meets because of this language barrier.

• Current drug testing continually effects a "cat-and-mouse" approach to solving the anabolic hormone issue in sports. Since the "cat" is a slow pursuer of the quicker "mouse," drug testing seems always to be behind the newer drugs and hormones used by athletes. In this manner, a common source for concern among testing officials is "are these athletes taking something which we can't detect?"

The aspect of the current drug testing program employed for major international sporting events, such as the 1984 Olympics, which is of perhaps the highest immediate concern is that it misleads the general public and sports fans. When I have questioned people about the fact that no United States Olympic athlete was officially found to be using drugs, most believed this meant "drug free." It was apparent that many people really feel that only other countries' athletes used drugs, since they were caught with them by current testing techniques *during* the 1984 Olympic Games. This misconception has covered up the truth about the anabolic hormone–using American athletes.

Conversations with Olympic athletes and hopefuls, and with the coaches of some of these athletes, letters from Olympic athletes, conversations with doctors involved with the official testing, and my own knowledge of the various theoretical and practical limits of the official testing employed, have led me to conclude that *many American athletes were taking anabolic hormones prior to and during the 1984 Olympic Games*. The major anabolic hormones used were low to moderate amounts of testosterone and human growth hormone, both of which are not detected by current limits and testing standards. A typical regimen believed to be used and to be subsequently tested "clean" is in two parts: the use of various anabolic steroids by men and women up until a few months prior to the Games, then switching to the use of testosterone in low to moderate amounts with or without concomitant human growth hormone use for the last few months.

American athletes are aware that it is possible to use testosterone for its physical and mental attributes and then test "clean." This is because testosterone is a hormone normally found within the body of men and women, and devising a test to determine which athletes are using additional testosterone is difficult to do since the normal ranges in humans vary so greatly. So, in order not to falsely accuse an athlete, testing ratios for testosterone and its normal metabolites have to be set extremely high—so high that, in effect, most athletes know they can use testosterone, and even testosterone and its tested metabolite, epitestosterone, and pass official urine drug testing.

American athletes also know that the use of human growth hormone cannot be determined by current testing. They know that medical scientists are busy trying to develop a plausible test for human growth hormone, but none seems likely soon. Therefore, some American athletes who believe that human growth hormone is a powerful anabolic hormone, actually used hGH during the 1984 Games. Estimates which have been given to me by the aforementioned sources range from 30 to 50 percent of the track and field team!

Let the sports fan and general public be aware that drug testing of athletes, even at its most technical levels, is strictly a PR effort. The elegant testing at the 1984 Olympic Summer Games still "missed" the moderate use of testosterone and the entire use of human growth hormone. Both of these anabolic hormones are thought to affect human athletic performance in many ways.

So far as the Olympics go, medical science now has four years to develop new testing procedures, right? Yes, but as history will reveal, the development of new anabolic hormones is well ahead of the testing technology, and for the 1988 Olympic Games, anabolic hormones likely to be used by athletes and "missed" by testing are the following hormones synthesized by recombinant-DNA techniques:

- human growth hormone, hGH

- growth hormone releasing hormone, GHRH

- leutinizing hormone releasing hormone, LHRH

- somatomedin-C, Sc.

This routine of too-late, too-little will probably continue to be part of national and international competitive athletics. And athletic American youths will continue to use anabolic hormones that medical science makes available to them, with barely a clue as to what they are actually doing to themselves.

The Fantasizing Child

For the first time in history, young children, who have always tended to fantasize about muscular human physiques, now know that their fantasies can come true. What these children are *unaware* of is that the imposing muscular body they wish for is a product of continued drug use (hormonal manipulation). From a January 1985 issue of *Time* magazine the following information about the television program "Masters of the Universe" was reported:

• Nine million youths (aged 4 to 7) watch the program weekly.

• $500 million retail sales for "He-Man" and other "Masters of the Universe" toys were reported for the 1984 Christmas season.

• "Masters of the Universe" led all video cassette sales in fall 1984.

Many of us grew up under the influence of "cowboys and Indians" and only comic books contained heroes with muscular physiques. There were no imposingly muscular bodies to emulate in real life. I was content with emulating my father, who was fit, but definitely not a "He-Man." In fact, as I grew, and athletics became my love, lifting weights was discouraged for most sports. It was claimed that large muscles adversely affected athletic skills in most sports.

But today, weight training is encouraged for most every sport and the "He-Man" walks the beaches and the shopping malls. He is the "bouncer" at the local "meet-and-greet" nightclub, he has his picture in all the sports magazines, and he lives right down the street. So, in a young boy's mind, he sees the reality of becoming a "He-Man" himself. What a difference the widespread use of anabolic steroids has made!

Also for the first time in history, what parents genetically give their children can be overshadowed by the black market anabolic hormone dealer in the local health club or by misguided physicians, or even by the child himself or herself. To me, this is terrifying but it represents a challenge. Sir William Osler said, "The physician's challenge is the curing of disease, educating the people in the laws of health...."

A Proposal for Effective Action

For any official sincerely wishing to halt as much as possible the widespread use of athletic performance–enhancing drugs, especially anabolic steroids and hormones, the following things must be considered:

• exposure of the anabolic steroid epidemic;

• disclosure to the general public and sports fan of the shortcomings of drug testing alone;

• publicity of the linkage between athletic violence with increased drug use;

• educating people about new anabolic hormone drugs and other drugs which lend themselves to athletic abuse;

• educating the general public about the "steroid charisma" afflicting our youth;

• determining that steroid and hormone use for athletic enhancement must be prohibited by federal law;

• requiring that future sports medicine investigations of certain kinds have mandatory and "spot" drug testing as part of their power, as otherwise the results are meaningless.

Although I am a believer in the free enterprise system, it seems to me that federal government control of some things is essential for the welfare of Americans. My proposal to solve the athletes and drugs problem requires the cooperation of one of the most powerful political machines on earth, the Food and Drug Administration.

The FDA must reclassify anabolic steroids, testosterone and related drugs and analogs under Schedule II, with a written diagnosis required for dispensing them.

The FDA must classify and reclassify *all* of the present and future anabolic and growth stimulating hormones synthesized by recombinant-DNA genetic engineering techniques as Schedule I or Schedule II, with a written diagnosis required for dispensing them.

The proper rate of research can be best assured as above. Under these schedules, theoretically, diseased persons who actually need the drugs can have a legal avenue to obtain them. Athletic use would not be legal, which to some extent overrides the moral and ethical arguments. Since the technology to synthesize these hormones is so specialized, control of these hormones is possible by controlling the few manufacturers.

Certain national sporting institutions or agencies must be empowered to employ "spot" urine testing of any competitive athlete participating in college and professional athletics. The terms of the athlete's contract must specifically allow for "spot" urine testing with short notice by the appropriate personnel. If the athlete refuses to take, or fails, the testing, the contract is void and professional and college athletic privileges are revoked.

Any formal sports medicine study involved with determining the "pros" and "cons" of various athletic training principles must be able to rule out drug use as a factor. Otherwise, the study is misleading and useless. This is another reason why mandatory and "spot" testing for drugs, by appropriate agencies, should take place.

A formal sports medicine committee must be established to determine the role of these anabolic/growth-stimulating hormones in treating athletic injuries and diseased states. These powerful drugs do have a role in sports medicine, but not as specific ergogenic aids. This formal sports medicine committee should be made up of doctors from various backgrounds — orthopedics, athletic medicine, endocrinology and diagnostically related fields — and not simply a selection of figureheads.

Drugs that are cleared for use must be dispensed in a controlled fashion.

Ordinary man is at the end of his tether. Only a small, highly adaptable minority of the species can possibly survive. The rest will not trouble about it, finding such opiates and consolations as they have a mind for. Let us then conclude this speculation about the final phase in the history of life, by surveying the modifications of the human type that are in progress to-day."

H.G. Wells,
The Mind at the End of Its Tether (1946)

All of the facets of modern medical science have made such an impact on humanity that it makes one wonder how mankind ever survived without "miracle drugs" and the like. And, in my opinion, shortly there will come a time when the majority of people will have sustained physical and/or mental changes due to the influence of powerful synthetic hormones or other drugs introduced by modern medicine. And in this manner, the minority of people who will still remain "unviolated" from this standpoint will be the only remaining nonhormonally manipulated species of human. But, whether this manipulation is for the ultimate improvement or ultimate demise of mankind is unknown to me.

This book serves two distinct purposes. First, it firmly entrenches in the mind of the reader that stepwise, profound study should always evaluate complex and powerful advances in the medical science fields. Second, this book serves as my answer to the proverbial question of "Doc, just what is your stance on anabolic steroids for athletes?"

Index

About the Author

William N. Taylor, M.D., the author of highly respected sports medicine books, is a member of the Alpha Omega Alpha Honor Medical Society. He completed his B.S. degree in chemistry at the University of West Florida in 1975 and his M.S. in chemical and polymer engineering at the University of Tennessee in 1976; he was employed with the B.F. Goodrich Chemical Company in Avon Lake, Ohio, as a research engineer before earning an M.D. degree from the University of Miami School of Medicine in 1981. He has been a practicing physician in Florida since 1982.

Dr. Taylor wrote *Anabolic Steroids and the Athlete* in 1982 (published by McFarland & Company, Inc.). His *Marathon Running: A Medical Science Handbook* (also McFarland, 1982) has been translated into Japanese and is an extensive summary of the exercise physiology and other parameters of the sport.

Dr. Taylor currently writes articles for a dozen sports magazines in various capacities. He is the sports medicine editor for *Muscle Digest* and *Powerlifting-USA* magazines. He serves as department editor for *Muscle & Fitness* magazine and as contributing editor for the *American Medical Joggers Association Newsletter*, *Strength & Health*, *Iron Man*, *Muscular Development* and other periodicals. He is a Fellow of the American College of Sports Medicine and an American Medical Joggers Association member; he serves as clinic advisor for the American Running & Fitness Association, and is an active member of the United States Powerlifting Federation Sports Medicine Committee.

During 1984, Dr. Taylor presented his expert advice on the topics of anabolic steroid and human growth hormone use by athletes in several medical and sports medicine meetings internationally. These included the Honolulu, Boston and London AMJA Marathon medical meetings, the American College of Sports Medicine Meeting in San Diego, and the National Strength & Conditioning Association's convention in Pittsburgh.

He is the finisher of 13 marathons, the last six with his wife, Susan. Together, they served as official Drug Officers utilizing the Olympic protocol at the 1984 Women's World Powerlifting Championships in Santa Monica, California. Together, they have also served as judges in bodybuilding contests. Dr. Taylor is instrumental in the formation of national policies that will determine the fate and direction of several aspects of drug use by athletes.